Budget Cookbook

3rd Edition

103 Delicious & Easy Recipes That Will CUT Your Grocery Bill in Half

Feed 4 for Under $10 A Meal

by Olivia Rogers

Copyright © 2017 By Olivia Rogers
All rights reserved. No part of this book may be reproduced in any form without permission in writing from the author. No part of this publication may be reproduced or transmitted in any form or by any means, mechanic, electronic, photocopying, recording, by any storage or retrieval system, or transmitted by email without the permission in writing from the author and publisher.
For information regarding permissions write to author at
Olivia@TheMenuAtHome.com
Reviewers may quote brief passages in review.

Please note that credit for the images used in this book go to the respective owners. You can view this at: TheMenuAtHome.com/image-list

Olivia Rogers
TheMenuAtHome.com

Table of Contents

Introduction _____ *7*
1. Veggie Quesadillas _____ *7*
2. Roast Chicken with Red Potato & Squash _____ *8*
3. Toasted BLT Sandwiches _____ *9*
4. Chicken, Rice, & Mushrooms _____ *9*
5. Heart Healthy Shrimp Salad _____ *10*
6. French Bread Pizzas _____ *12*
7. Turkey Patties _____ *13*
8. Salmon & Brown Rice _____ *14*
9. Chicken Parma _____ *15*
10. Chickpea Burgers _____ *16*
11. Salami and Stuffed Shells _____ *17*
12. Gnocchi & Zucchini _____ *18*
13. Texas Chili _____ *18*
14. Honey Soy & Ginger Chicken Wings _____ *19*
15. Rosemary & Apricot Tenderloins _____ *20*
16. Margarita Pizza _____ *21*
17. Butternut Squash & Chicken Soup _____ *22*
18. Veggie, Avo, & White Bean Burritos _____ *22*
19. Mustard Seed Chicken _____ *23*
20. Turkey Meatball Subs _____ *24*
21. Beer Braised Beef _____ *25*
22. Easy Spinach Cheddar Quiche _____ *26*
23. Mediterranean Tomato Chickpea Salad _____ *27*
24. Greek Pasta _____ *28*
25. Spaghetti Squash with Chicken _____ *29*

26. Cauliflower Chickpea Curry _____ 30
27. Beef Stroganoff _____ 31
28. Taco Casserole _____ 31
29. Twice Baked Bacon and Cheddar Potatoes _____ 32
30. Stuffed Tomatoes _____ 33
31. Tomato Ricotta Crustini with Chicken _____ 34
32. Spinach Sausage Egg Casserole _____ 35
33. Curry Chicken Salad _____ 35
34. Philly Cheesesteak Sandwiches _____ 36
35. Fish Tacos _____ 37
36. Turkey Chili _____ 38
37. Homemade Chicken and Veggie Soup _____ 39
38. Ranch Pasta Salad with Chicken _____ 40
39. Sweet Potato Patties _____ 40
40. Sun Dried Tomato Chicken _____ 41
41. Stuffed Peppers _____ 42
42. Chicken Broccoli Pie _____ 43
43. Italian Chicken Casserole _____ 44
44. Chicken Fried Rice _____ 45
45. Mexican Baked Potatoes _____ 45
46. Southwest Style Rice and Beans _____ 46
47. Chicken and Broccoli Tetrazzini _____ 47
48. Easy Taco Salad _____ 48
49. Stuffed Zucchini _____ 48
50. Sausage Potatoes and Peppers _____ 49
51. Baked Ziti _____ 50
52. Green Beans in Coconut Milk _____ 51

53. Minestrone Soup with Macaroni _____ 52

54. Chili Beans with Pasta _____ 53

55. Tuna Spaghetti with Tomatoes and Garlic _____ 54

56. Beef and Vegetable Stew _____ 55

57. Garlic-Herb Beef Roast _____ 56

58. Paella in A Flash _____ 57

59. Baked Mushroom-Chicken Curry Rice _____ 58

60. Red Rice Soup with Beef _____ 60

61. Stir-fried Shrimp Hofan _____ 61

62. Corned Beef Hearty Soup _____ 62

63. Meatloaf Pasta Parmigiana _____ 63

64. Luncheon Meat Katsudon _____ 64

65. Seafood Fried Rice _____ 66

66. Cajun Pork Chops with Gravy _____ 67

67. Chicken Barbecue with Java Rice _____ 68

68. Egg and Spinach Sandwiches _____ 69

69. Roast Chicken with Potatoes and Butternut Squash _____ 70

70. Chicken and Rice with Broccoli _____ 71

71. Chipotle Chicken Casserole _____ 72

72. Turkey Sausage Mushroom and Potato Gratin _____ 74

73. Chicken Focaccia Sandwich Recipe _____ 75

74. Ginger Turkey Stir Fry _____ 76

75. Potato Crusted Chicken Fingers _____ 77

76. Ham Casserole _____ 78

77. Shredded Pork Tacos _____ 79

78. Maple Chili Gazed Pork Medallions _____ 80

79. Maple Brined Pork _____ 81

80. Slow Cooker Pulled Pork _____ 82
81. Cornmeal Crusted Pork _____ 83
82. Grilled Pork with Pineapple _____ 84
83. Crockpot Chili _____ 85
84. Classic Meatloaf _____ 86
85. Asian Beef Steak Noodles _____ 87
86. Sloppy Joe Bake _____ 88
87. Quick Beef Stir Fry _____ 89
88. Classic Pastie Slab _____ 90
89. Picadillo _____ 91
90. Classic Tuna Macaroni Salad _____ 92
91. Shrimp, Avocado and Grapefruit Salad _____ 93
92. Korean Fish Stir Fry _____ 94
93. Seafood Skewers _____ 95
94. Tuna Noodle Casserole _____ 96
95. White Fish Baked with Lemon Thyme and Garlic _____ 97
96. Fettuccine Seafood Alfredo _____ 98
97. Roasted Mushroom and Lentil Soup _____ 99
98. Sour Cream and Chives Pasta _____ 100
99. Black Eyed Peas and Greens _____ 101
100. Potato and Broccoli Casserole _____ 102
101. Vegetarian Tacos _____ 103
102. Parmigiana Allai Melanzane (Eggplant Bake) _____ 104
103. 5-Ingredient Power Casserole _____ 105
Final Words _____ 106
Disclaimer _____ 107

Introduction

Cooking for the whole family is a challenging task. Planning and keeping it healthy and delicious while being under a strict budget is difficult especially if you have young kids at home. When you are cooking in a daily basis, it is hard to actually have a variation with your cooking. Thus, to prevent your family from getting bored with the same meals that you are cooking for them, you have to make sure you offer them different kinds of meal.

In these days and time, it is hard to cook up complicated meals all the time, maybe save all the prestige recipes for the weekends and cook up easy and affordable recipes during the weekdays. In that way you will be able to prevent your family from getting bored.

If you are worrying that you might not be able to find easy and affordable recipes, don't worry! In this book, allow me to show you quick, delicious and affordable meals that your family will surely enjoy. Learn from different techniques and explore different flavors from different parts of the world that would excite your palate. Add a few know-hows from simple tips given that would make your cooking fun and enjoyable. So, read on and step into the wonderful world of cooking. Make your life simple. Enjoy and try out these exciting recipes! Happy cooking!

1. Veggie Quesadillas

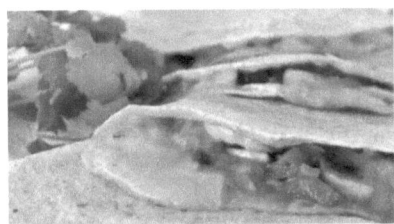

Ingredients

- ½ chopped red bell pepper
- 1 medium purple onion
- 1 deseeded and chopped jalapeno (can leave seeds in)
- 6-inch whole wheat or spinach tortillas
- ½ cup shredded Monterey jack cheese
- 1 small chopped tomato
- Light dairy sour cream (optional
- Cilantro and juice from a lime (optional)

Method

1. In a bowl combine bell pepper, onion, jalapeno, tomato, cilantro, and lime juice. Toss to form the veggie filling. In a greased pan on medium heat, place a tortilla and quickly spoon a portion of the veggie filling onto half of the tortilla. Sprinkle cheese on top of the filling.

2. Allow to cook until the cheese is slightly melted, and fold the empty tortilla half on top of the filling to form a half moon shape. Flip tortilla and cook until tortilla is slightly brown. Cut into 3 triangles and serve with sour cream.

2. Roast Chicken with Red Potato & Squash

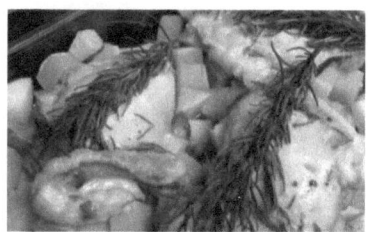

Ingredients

- 1 ½ tsp minced garlic
- McCormick's Rotisserie Chicken Seasoning (or seasoning of choice)
- 1 3lb roasting chicken (cleaned & giblets/neck removed and discarded)
- Red potatoes (cleaned and halved)
- Butternut squash (cleaned and cubed)
- 1 tsp low fat butter (melted)
- ½ tsp salt and pepper

Method

1. Preheat oven to 400F. In a small bowl, combine garlic, butter, salt, and pepper. Starting at the neck, loosen skin from breast and drumsticks by pushing your fingers between the skin and the meat. Rub garlic mixture under loosened skin, and sprinkle McCormick's Rotisserie Seasoning all over chicken.

2. Place chicken breast side up in broiler pan, and arrange potatoes and squash around chicken. Bake in oven for 1 hour, or until meat is 165F. Let meat stand for 10 minutes before carving.

3. Toasted BLT Sandwiches

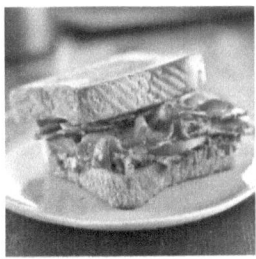

Ingredients

- 1 red onion sliced
- Butter
- Shredded reduced-fat sharp white cheddar cheese
- Wheat bread
- Fresh cos lettuce leaves
- 1 sliced fresh tomato
- Center-cut bacon
- Mayonnaise (optional)

Method

1. Cook bacon and lay on paper towels to absorb as much grease as possible. Butter a slice of wheat bread and place butter side down in a pan on medium heat. Quickly add onion, mayo, cheese, tomato, and bacon to the bread. Butter another slice of wheat bread and place butter side up on top of the stack.

2. Once bread is lightly toasted and golden brown, flip the stack carefully. Once that bead is lightly toasted, remove sandwich from heat, add cos lettuce (if you add on stove the lettuce will become mushy not nice and crisp) to sandwich, and enjoy.

4. Chicken, Rice, & Mushrooms

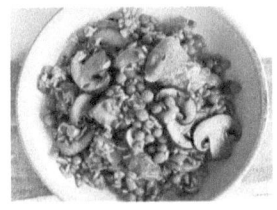

Ingredients

- 2 cups boiling water
- ¼ cup dried porcini mushrooms
- 1lbs chicken breast (cleaned and cubed)
- 1 tsp sweet paprika
- Salt
- Ground black pepper
- ¾ cup chopped onion
- 8oz cremini mushrooms, sliced
- ¾ cup uncooked brown basmati rice
- 2 cups green peas
- 1 tbsp. chopped fresh thyme

Method

1. In a bowl combine, boiling water and mushrooms. Set aside for 20 minutes, drain (save liquid), and chop mushrooms. Season chicken cubes with paprika, salt, and pepper to taste. In a large greased (olive oil) pan on medium heat, sauté chicken for 5 minutes, and remove from chicken from pan. Using the same pan add onion, cremini mushrooms, and ¼ tsp salt and ground black pepper. Sauté for 4 minutes.

2. Stir in the saved porcini liquid, chopped porcini, and rice. Bring to a boil. Once boiling, cover and reduce the heat. Allow to simmer for 35 minutes. Stir in the chicken, peas, and thyme. Cover and cook 10 minutes.

5. Heart Healthy Shrimp Salad

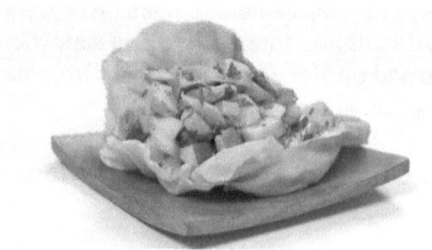

Ingredients

- Olive oil
- 12oz peeled medium shrimp
- Salt

- Freshly ground black pepper
- 1 peeled and cubed grapefruit (save juice)
- 2 tbsp. chopped fresh tarragon
- 2 tsp brown sugar
- 1 tsp chopped shallot
- 6 cups chopped romaine lettuce
- 1 peeled and sliced avocado

Method

1. Grease pan with olive oil, and on medium heat add shrimp, salt, and pepper to taste. Cook for 3 minutes or until shrimp are done, and remove from heat.

2. In a bowl combine grapefruit juice, 2 tbsp. oil, ¼ tsp salt, ⅛ tsp pepper, tarragon, brown sugar, and shallots. Stir well with a whisk. To the same bowl add lettuce and toss. Top each serving with avocado, shrimp, and grapefruit.

Read This FIRST - 100% FREE BONUS

FOR A LIMITED TIME ONLY – Get Olivia's best-selling book *"The #1 Cookbook: Over 170+ of the Most Popular Recipes Across 7 Different Cuisines!"* absolutely FREE!

Readers have absolutely loved this book because of the wide variety of recipes. It is highly recommended you check these recipes out and see what you can add to your home menu!

Once again, as a big thank-you for downloading this book, I'd like to offer it to you *100% FREE for a LIMITED TIME ONLY!*

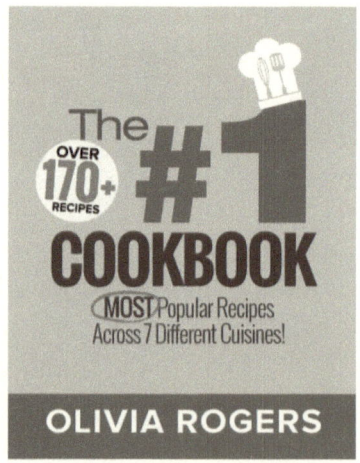

Get your free copy at:

TheMenuAtHome.com/Bonus

6. French Bread Pizzas

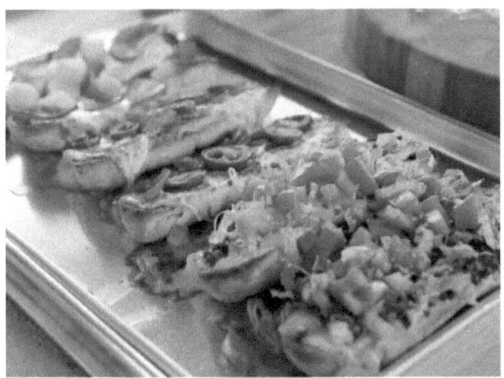

Ingredients

- 1 fresh loaf of French bread
- Lower-sodium marinara sauce
- Cubed pepperoni
- Part-skim mozzarella cheese
- 1 sliced purple onion
- 1 chopped green pepper
- Any other toppings of choice

Method

1. Preheat oven to 350F. Take French bread and slice down center to form 2 halves. On each half spread marinara sauce (not too much for it can make the bread soggy instead of crunchy), and add cheese, onion, pepperoni, and pepper toppings. Place halves directly on the oven rack and bake until cheese is melted and bread is toasted. Allow to cool before serving.

7. Turkey Patties

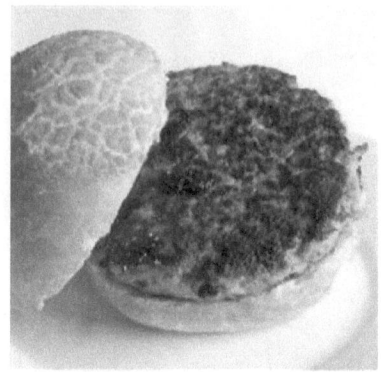

Ingredients

- 1lbs turkey mince
- 1 finely chopped lemongrass stalk
- 2 tbsp. minced garlic
- Juice of a lime
- 3 tbsp. low-sodium soy sauce
- Chopped fresh coriander
- 1 chopped red chili
- 1 egg
- ½ cup bread crumbs

Method

1. In a bowl, add turkey, lemongrass, garlic, lime juice, soy sauce, coriander, chili, egg, and bread crumbs. Mix together using your hands. Shape into patties. In a greased pan on medium heat cook the turkey patties until cooked throughout. Allow to set for 5 minutes before serving.

8. Salmon & Brown Rice

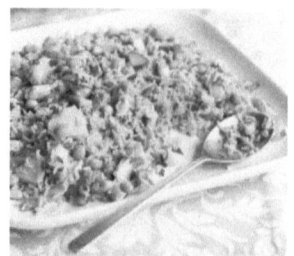

Ingredients

- ½ lbs. brown basmati rice
- ¼ lbs. frozen soya beans, defrosted
- 2 salmon fillets
- 1 chopped cucumber
- Chopped small bunch spring onions
- Chopped fresh coriander
- Juice of 1 lime
- 1 chopped red chili
- 4 tsp low sodium soy sauce

Method

1. In a pan on medium heat boil rice for 8 minutes until fully cooked and drain. The last 2 minutes add the soya beans to the rice. Place the salmon fillets on a plate and microwave for 3 minutes. If the salmon isn't fully cooked add on another 30 seconds until done. Remove the skin from the fillet, and shred.

2. Carefully mix the cucumber, spring onions, coriander and salmon into the rice and beans. Before serving sprinkle soy sauce, chili, and lime juice.

9. Chicken Parma

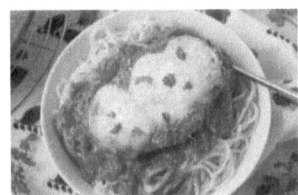

Ingredients

- 2 large, skinless chicken breasts, halved through the middle
- 2 eggs, beaten
- ⅓ cup breadcrumbs
- ⅓ cup grated parmesan cheese
- 1 tbsp. olive oil
- 2 tsp minced garlic
- 1 ½ cup tomato puree
- 1 tsp sugar

- 1 tsp dried oregano
- Half a 125g ball light mozzarella, torn

Method

1. Dip chicken breast in egg, and roll in breadcrumbs mixed with ⅙ cup parmesan cheese. In a medium size pan heat the olive oil, and sauté garlic for 1 minute. Then add the tomato puree, sugar, and oregano. Season and simmer for 5-10 minutes. Preheat oven to 350F.

2. Heat grill to a high heat and cook the chicken for 5 minutes. Pour the tomato sauce into a shallow ovenproof dish and add the chicken. Sprinkle over the mozzarella and remaining Parmesan and bake for 5-8 minutes until cheese has melted and sauce is bubbling.

10. Chickpea Burgers

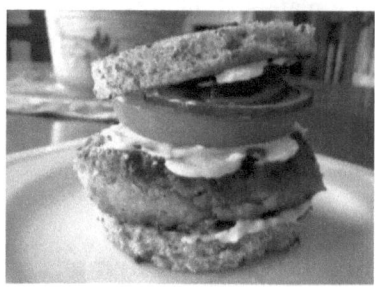

Ingredients

- 1 can chickpeas, drained
- Zest of a lemon
- Juice of ½ a lemon
- 1 tsp ground cumin
- Chopped coriander
- 1 egg
- ⅔ cup breadcrumbs
- ½ purple onion diced
- 1 tbsp. olive oil
- 4 small whole wheat buns
- Tomato, cucumber, purple onion, and chili sauce (suggested toppings)

Method

1. In a bowl, beat chickpeas, lemon zest, lemon juice, cumin, half the coriander, egg, and some seasoning. Add to the mixture ⅔ cup of breadcrumbs and diced onions.

2. Form 4 burger patties. Heat oil in a pan on medium heat. Cook burgers on each side for 5 minutes keeping in mind that they don't burn. Top burgers with suggested toppings in ingredients on whole wheat buns.

11. Salami and Stuffed Shells

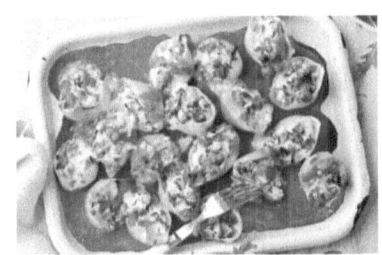

Ingredients

- Large dried jumbo pasta shells
- ½ lb. chopped shaved mild salami
- ½ sliced red onion
- 6 cups tomato puree
- 1 tub ricotta cheese
- 2 ½ cups grated pizza cheese
- ½ cup fresh basil leaves, shredded
- 2 tsp olive oil

Method

1. Preheat oven to 390F. In a medium pot, bring water seasoned with salt to a boil. Add shells to water, cook for 8-10 minutes or until soft, rinse with cold water, and drain. Heat oil in a pan over medium heat, and add salami and onion. Sauté for 5 minutes or until onion has softened and salami is golden. Remove from heat.

2. Pour tomato puree over base of a baking dish. In a bowl, combine salami mixture, ricotta, 2 cups cheese, and basil and mix well. Carefully spoon portions of this mixture into each pasta shell. Arrange shells in prepared dish (shell opening facing up). Sprinkle with extra cheese. Bake for 20 minutes or until cheese is melted.

12. Gnocchi & Zucchini

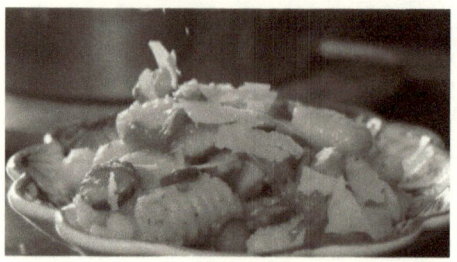

Ingredients

- 1 lbs. gnocchi
- 2 tbsp. butter
- 2 chopped shallots
- 1 lbs. zucchini (sliced thin)
- pint cherry tomatoes (cut in half)
- ½ tsp salt
- ¼ tsp nutmeg
- Ground pepper
- ½ cup parmesan cheese
- ½ cup chopped fresh parsley

Method

1. In a medium pot, bring water seasoned with salt to a boil. Add gnocchi to water, cook for 8-10 minutes or until soft, rinse with cold water, and drain.

2. In a large pan on medium heat melt butter and add shallots and zucchini. Cook and stir often, until softened. Add tomatoes, salt, nutmeg and pepper to pan. Cook about 1 to 2 minutes, and then stir in parmesan and parsley. Add the gnocchi to pan and, toss to coat. Enjoy!

13. Texas Chili

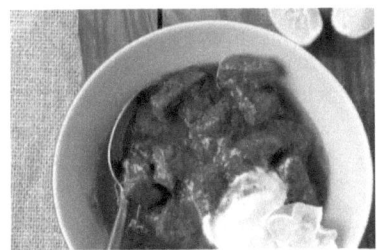

Ingredients

- 1 pound 93%-lean ground beef
- 1 large red bell pepper, chopped
- 1 large onion, chopped
- 6 cloves garlic, chopped
- 1 tablespoon chili powder
- 2 teaspoons ground cumin
- 1/4 teaspoon cayenne pepper, or to taste
- 1 16-ounce jar green salsa, green enchilada sauce or taco sauce
- 1/4 cup water
- 1 15-ounce can pinto or kidney beans, rinsed

Method

1. In a large pan on medium heat cook beef, bell pepper, and onion until meat is browned. Add garlic, chili powder, cumin, water, salsa, and cayenne to the pan and bring to a simmer. Reduce heat, cover, and cook for about 10 to 15 minutes. Stir in beans and cook for 1 minute. Serve and enjoy.

14. Honey Soy & Ginger Chicken Wings

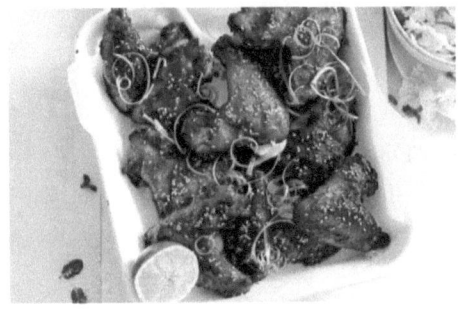

Ingredients

- 25 chicken wings
- Ginger and honey marinade
- 5 finely chopped spring onions
- 5 tbsp. honey
- 2 tbsp. soy sauce
- 1 sliced red chili
- 1 tbsp. of fresh grated ginger
- 4-5 sprigs of thyme

Method

1. In a bowl, add ginger and honey marinade, onions, honey, soy sauce, red chili, ginger, and thyme and mix well. Lay chicken wings in a shallow dish, and pour the marinade over the wings. Cover and place in the fridge for 24 hours. Heat your barbecue until hot, and cook for 15–20 minutes while turning, until cooked through.

15. Rosemary & Apricot Tenderloins

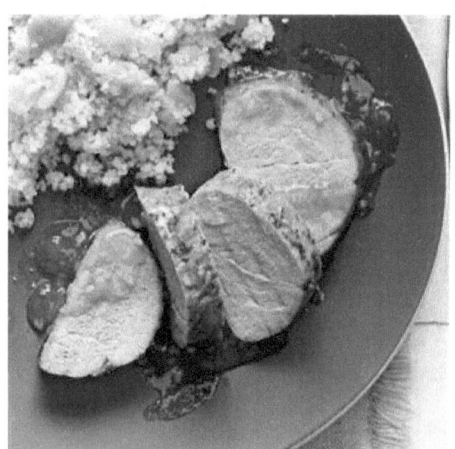

Ingredients

- 1 tbsp. country Dijon mustard
- 1 tbsp. apricot fruit spread
- 1 lbs. pork tenderloin
- ⅓ cup chopped apricots
- 1 tbsp. rosemary

Method

1. Preheat the oven to 450 degrees F. In a bowl, add mustard and fruit spread, and microwave until spread is soft. Make a lengthwise cut in tenderloin, and spread half the mustard mixture in the pork loin. Top with apricots and sprinkle with half the rosemary.

2. Tie the roast closed with cooking string and place it seam side down on the greased baking sheet. Pour the remaining mustard mixture over the outside of the pork and sprinkle with the remaining rosemary. Bake in the oven 24 minutes.

16. Margarita Pizza

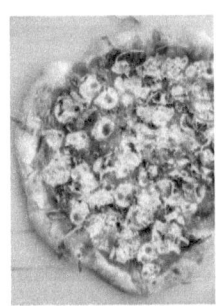

Ingredients

- Onion flakes
- 1 large tomato sliced thin
- Low-fat mozzarella cheese
- Parmesan cheese
- Fresh basil
- Extra virgin olive oil
- Oregano

Method

1. Preheat the oven to 400F. Knead the dough to work out any bubbles, while dusting your hands with flour. Place dough in a pan greased lightly, and press in the minced garlic throughout the dough.

2. Sprinkle base with onion flakes, parmesan cheese, and oregano. Place sliced tomato and mozzarella on top. Garnish the top with the fresh basil. Cook 15-20 minutes or until base is golden brown

17. Butternut Squash & Chicken Soup

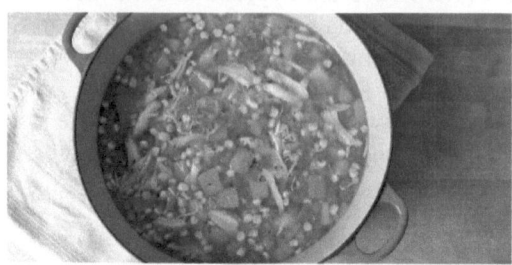

Ingredients

- Diced onion
- 1 butternut squash cubed
- 4 cups low-sodium chicken broth
- 2-3 boneless and skinless chicken breasts cubed
- Salt and pepper
- 2-3 tbsp. olive oil
- ¼ tsp coriander
- ¼ tsp cumin

Method

1. Place onion, squash, and chicken on a baking tray tossed with the olive oil, and salt and pepper to taste. Roast until chicken is cooked through and squash is tender.

2. Scrape onion, chicken, and squash into a pot. Add broth and spices then bring to a simmer. Mash up some of the squash pieces. Continue to simmer for 10-15 minutes so soup will thicken. Season with salt and pepper to taste.

18. Veggie, Avo, & White Bean Burritos

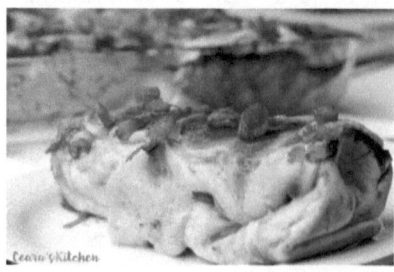

Ingredients

- 2 tbsp. cider vinegar
- 1 tbsp. canola oil
- 2 tsp canned chipotle chile in adobo sauce, finely chopped
- ¼ tsp salt
- 2 cups shredded red cabbage
- 1 medium carrot, shredded
- ¼ cup chopped cilantro
- 1 can white beans
- 1 avocado
- ½ cup shredded Cheddar cheese
- 2 tbsp. finely chopped red onion
- 4 whole-wheat tortillas

Method

1. In a bowl, whisk vinegar, oil, chipotle chile, and salt in a medium bowl. Add cabbage, carrot and cilantro and toss. Mash beans and avocado in another medium bowl. Stir in cheese and onion. Spread bean-avocado mixture onto a tortilla, top with cabbage-carrot slaw, and roll.

19. Mustard Seed Chicken

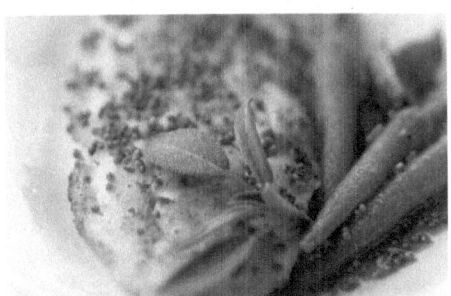

Ingredients

- 4 chicken breasts
- 2 tbsp. mustard seed
- 2 zucchinis, sliced thin
- 2 banana peppers, make sure they're sweet
- 2 shallots sliced
- 1 ½ cups halved cherry tomatoes
- 4 tsp olive oil

- 1 tbsp. chopped fresh thyme
- ½ tsp salt
- ¼ tsp ground pepper

Method

1. Pre-heat your oven to approximately 400F. Make a pocket with aluminum foil, by folding the foil in half and pinching together on the ends. Spread chicken breast with mustard seed and place in the foil packet.

2. Toss into a large bowl, the following, tomatoes, zucchini, shallots, thyme, oil, peppers, and of course, salt and pepper. Pour the mixture into the packet, and gently shake bag to mix up.

3. Close the packet very simply by folding over the top. Place the packet on a baking sheet, and start baking until the point where the vegetables become tender, as well as the chicken is cooked through out, this should take approximately 25 minutes.

20. Turkey Meatball Subs

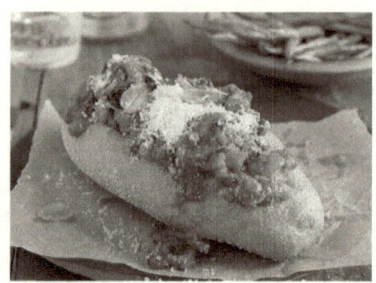

Ingredients

- 1 ¼ lbs. minced turkey
- ½ cup breadcrumbs
- 2 tbsp. chopped onion
- 1 tbsp. chopped parsley
- ½ cup parmesan cheese
- salt and pepper to taste
- 1 tsp minced garlic
- 1 tsp fennel seeds
- 1 egg
- zest of half a lemon

- 3 tbsp. olive oil
- 1 can pizza sauce
- 4 ounces fresh mozzarella, sliced

Method

1. Preheat oven to 400F. In a large bowl, by hands, gently mix together minced turkey, bread crumbs, onion, parsley, parmesan, salt and pepper, garlic, fennel seed, egg, and lemon zest. Shape into balls, and place on a foil-lined baking sheet.

2. In a small bowl, mix one spoonful of your pizza sauce with olive oil, and brush on top of each meatball. Bake for 15 minutes. Remove meatballs from oven, spoon sauce on top of meatballs, and cover each with a slice of cheese. Broil another 3 to 5 minutes until cheese is bubbly and golden. Remove meatballs and serve.

21. Beer Braised Beef

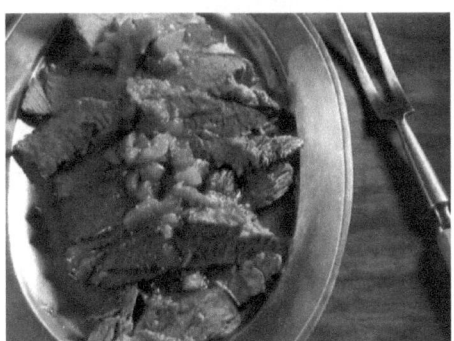

Ingredients

- 3 tbsp. flour
- 1 ½ tbsp. oil
- 1 boneless chuck roast
- 1 tsp salt
- ½ tsp black pepper
- 1 cup beef broth
- 4 tbsp. minced garlic
- 1 12oz dark beer
- 1 bay leaf
- 3 carrots, peeled and cubed
- 9 oz. small turnips, peeled and cubed

- 1 medium onion, peeled and sliced
- ¼ cup chopped fresh parsley

Method

1. Preheat oven to 300F. Heat oil in a pot oven over medium-high heat. Season beef evenly on all sides with salt and pepper and coat in flour. Add beef to pan and cook for 10 minutes, turning to brown on all sides.

2. Add broth, garlic, beer, and bay leaf to pan while scraping pan to remove browned bits. Bring to a boil then cover and bake at 300F for 1 ½ hours. Add carrots, cover, and cook 25 minutes. Add ½ teaspoon salt, turnips, and onion cover and cook an additional 1 hour or until vegetables are tender and beef.

22. Easy Spinach Cheddar Quiche

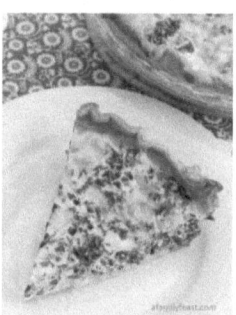

Ingredients

- 2 cups of milk or cream
- 4 large eggs
- ¾ cup of biscuit baking mixture or self-rising flour
- ¼ cup softened butter or margarine
- 1 cup of grated Parmesan cheese
- 1 package of frozen spinach or 1 cup of dices fresh spinach
- 1 cup of cubed sausage or ham
- 8 ounces of shredded Cheddar cheese

Method

1. Preheat oven to 375 degrees. Lightly grease a 10-inch pie pan or a medium sized baking dish.

2. In a large mixing bowl whisk the eggs and milk together. Stir in the baking mix. butter and parmesan cheese. Batter will be lumpy. Stir in the sausage or ham and Cheddar cheese. Pour into prepared pie pan or baking dish.

3. Bake uncovered in preheated oven for 50 minutes, until eggs are set and top is golden brown.

23. Mediterranean Tomato Chickpea Salad

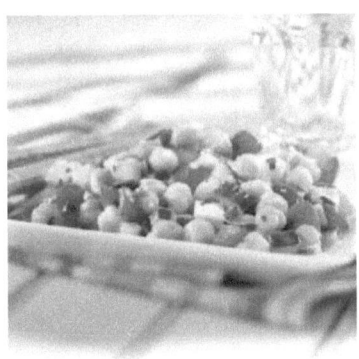

Ingredients

- 12-ounce package of grape tomatoes
- 15.5 ounce can of chickpeas/garbanzo beans
- 6 oz. package of crumbled Feta cheese
- 2 tablespoons of Extra Virgin Olive Oil
- 1-2 tablespoons of Black Pepper (or to taste)
- 1 tablespoon of salt (or to taste)
- 2 tablespoons of fresh Dill (or to taste)

Method

1. Wash the tomatoes and cut them in half. Place them to the side in a large bowl. Drain and rinse the chickpeas/garbanzo beans. Remove the hulls.

2. Toss the chickpeas/garbanzo beans with the tomatoes. Add the olive oil and the spices. Mix so that the tomatoes and chickpeas are coated. Mix in the Feta cheese. Refrigerate for at least two hours and serve. Delicious alone or served with baked chicken. Also, fantastic stuffed into a pita for a quick lunch.

24. Greek Pasta

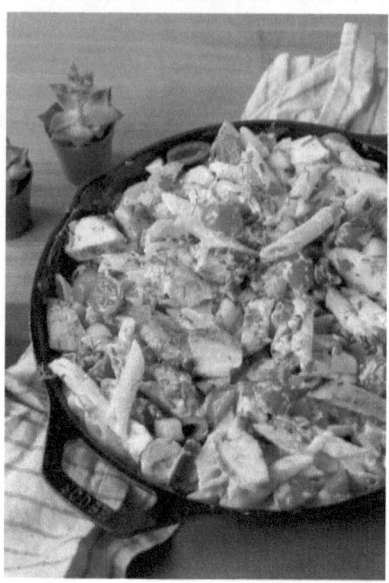

Ingredients

- 3 large tomatoes, cut into wedges or two 12-ounce cans of sliced tomatoes
- 2 tablespoons olive oil
- 1/4 teaspoon salt
- Freshly ground black pepper
- 15 ounces can of Cannellini beans
- 1/2 pound of penne pasta or bowtie pasta
- 1/4 cup fresh basil leaves, torn
- 2 tablespoons of grated Parmesan cheese

Method

1. Wash and slice the tomatoes if using fresh tomatoes. Combine the tomatoes and the Cannellini beans in a medium saucepan. Do not drain the Cannellini beans. Heat through then simmer. Season to taste.

2. Cook the pasta according to the directions on the package. Drain well. Spoon the tomatoes and Cannellini beans over the hot pasta. Top with fresh basil leaves and grated Parmesan cheese. To make a heartier meal serve baked chicken breast with the pasta.

25. Spaghetti Squash with Chicken

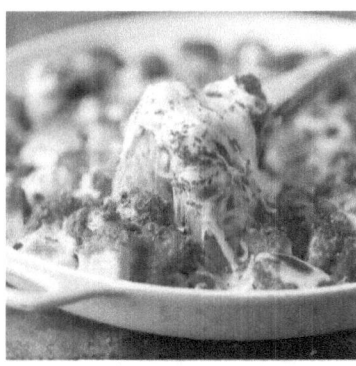

Ingredients

- 1 large Spaghetti squash
- 4 chicken breasts
- 1 16-ounce jar of tomato sauce
- 1 cup of shredded Mozzarella cheese
- 2 tablespoons olive oil
- Salt and pepper to taste

Method

1. Preheat the oven to 400 degrees. Coat the chicken breasts with olive oil. Add salt and pepper. Place the chicken breasts on a baking sheet and bake them at 400 degrees for 30 minutes or until the center is cooked through.

2. Cut the Spaghetti squash in half lengthwise. Place each half with the cut side facing up in a baking dish with a shallow layer of water in the bottom of the dish. Bake uncovered for 30-40 minutes in the oven with the chicken.

3. Remove both the chicken and the squash from the oven. Let the chicken rest. Using a fork pull all the strands of squash from the rind. The strands will look like cooked spaghetti and should pull away from the rind easily. Plate the squash the way you would plate spaghetti.

4. Heat the tomato sauce in a saucepan. Slice the chicken into thick slices while the sauce heats. Place chicken slices on top of the spaghetti squash and top with tomato sauce and Mozzarella cheese.

26. Cauliflower Chickpea Curry

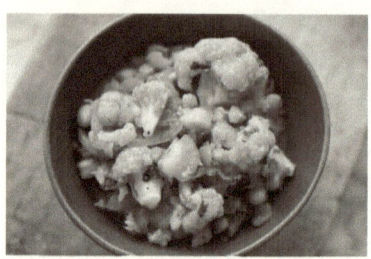

Ingredients

- 1 tablespoon vegetable oil or olive oil
- 2 teaspoons of yellow curry powder
- 1 medium yellow onion, sliced
- 1 tablespoon of ginger
- 15.5 ounce can of chickpeas/garbanzo beans
- 1 head cauliflower, cored, florets separated or one 12-ounce package of frozen cauliflower
- 15-ounce can of whole, peeled tomatoes
- 1 teaspoon Kosher salt
- 1/8 teaspoon freshly ground black pepper
- 1/2 cup water
- 1/2 cup roughly chopped cilantro
- 2 teaspoons minced fresh mint leaves
- 1 cup of white or jasmine rice

Method

1. In a large pot or deep skillet pour the oil and let it heat up. Add the curry powder. When that mixture is hot, add the onions and let them cook down until tender, about 8 minutes usually.

2. Add the ginger and the chickpeas to the mixture and let it heat through. Add the tomatoes, shredding them into chunks with your fingers. Add the tomato juice from the can as well.

3. Add the cauliflower and the water to the mixture and let it all heat up together. Bring just to a boil then cover and simmer for about 15 minutes. While the curry is simmering prepare the rice according to the directions. Remove from heat and add the cilantro and mint. Serve over rice.

27. Beef Stroganoff

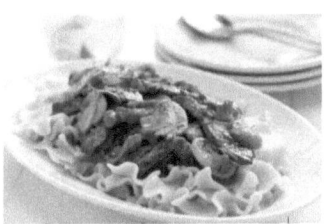

Ingredients

- 1 pound of lean ground beef
- 16-ounce package of wide egg noodles
- 12 ounces can of cream of mushroom condensed soup
- 16-ounce package of sour cream
- 1 teaspoon of salt
- 1 teaspoon of black pepper
- 1 diced onion
- ½ clove of garlic, diced

Method

1. In a large skillet brown the ground beef. Add in the onions and garlic and simmer. While the meat, onions and garlic are simmering prepare the egg noodles.

2. Add the condensed soup to the meat, onions and garlic and mix well. Simmer for about 10 minutes or until heated through. Drain the egg noodles when they are done and plate them.

3. Add the sour cream to the ground beef mixture and mix well. Cover and simmer until the sour cream is heated through. Salt and pepper to taste. Pour the ground beef mixture over the egg noodles and serve.

28. Taco Casserole

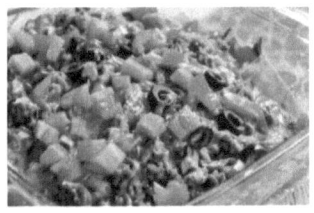

Ingredients

- 1 pound of lean ground beef
- 1 package of taco seasoning
- 8-ounce jar of taco sauce
- 16-ounce bag of tortilla chips
- 2 cups of shredded Mexican blend cheese or shredded Cheddar cheese
- 12-ounce container of sour cream
- 12-ounce can of diced tomatoes

Method

1. In a skillet brown the ground beef. Mix in the taco seasoning and simmer for about 10 minutes. While the beef is simmering preheat the oven to 375 degrees.

2. Line the bottom of a large baking dish or a casserole pan with tortilla chips. Pour the beef mixture on top. Add the tomatoes and the taco sauce. Add one cup of the cheese.

3. Place a layer of tortilla chips on top. Add the second cup of cheese on the top of the tortilla chips. Bake at 375 degrees for 15-20 minutes. Serve with sour cream.

29. Twice Baked Bacon and Cheddar Potatoes

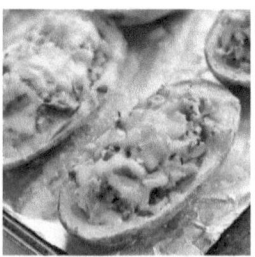

Ingredients

- 4 russet potatoes
- 1 cup chopped bacon
- 1/2 cup milk
- 2–3 tablespoons of shredded Cheddar cheese
- Salt and pepper, to taste
- 2 tablespoons of olive oil

Method

1. Preheat oven to 425 degrees. Scrub potatoes, then poke each several times with a fork. Brush them with olive oil. Place the potatoes on a baking tray, and bake for 50-60 minutes or until tender. Once cooked, remove from the oven.

2. Slice potatoes lengthwise, and scoop the insides out into a blender, leaving a good 1/4 inch of potato flesh still attached to the potato skin. Add the bacon and milk to the potato in the blender and blend until smooth.

3. Season to taste with salt and pepper. Scoop the pureed bacon and potato mixture back into the potato skins. Sprinkle with the grated cheddar cheese, return to the baking sheet, and bake for another 10 minutes.

30. Stuffed Tomatoes

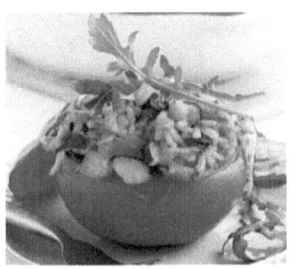

Ingredients

- 4 large tomatoes
- 1 cup of crumbled Feta cheese or 1 cup of a cheese of your choice
- 1 handful of parsley
- 1 tablespoon olive oil
- Salt and pepper to taste

Method

1. Preheat the oven to 400 degrees. Wash the tomatoes. Slice the tops off of each tomato about 1/2-inch down from the top of each stem, making a cap. Set the caps aside. Using a spoon, scoop out the inside flesh of each tomato, being careful not to pierce the skin. Lightly grease a glass baking dish with a bit of olive oil, and arrange the hollowed tomatoes (spaced evenly) with the sliced sides up.

2. Chop the parsley and mix with the crumbled feta or whatever cheese you want to use. Stuff each tomato with the cheese and parsley mixture. Season the tops of the stuffed tomatoes with salt and pepper and drizzle with olive oil.

3. Place the caps back on top of each tomato and bake for about 10 minutes, or until the tomatoes soften and begin to look shriveled and the cheese is melted.

31. Tomato Ricotta Crustini with Chicken

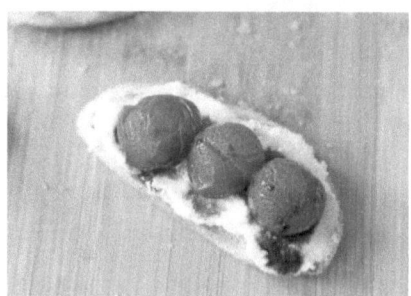

Ingredients

- 4-6 Roma tomatoes
- 4 large rolls like sandwich or sub rolls. Or flatbread.
- 16-ounce container of Ricotta cheese
- Salt and pepper to taste
- 2 cups sliced, cooked chicken breast. These can be leftovers or fresh.

Method

1. If you have some leftover chicken breasts this is a great way to use them up. Or you can buy pre-cooked chicken breasts or bake some. If you are baking chicken breasts bake them on a baking sheet at 400 degrees for 30 minutes. Let them cool slightly then slice them.

2. Preheat the oven to 375 degrees. Slice the tomatoes. Place the rolls with the flat side up on a baking sheet. Put 1-2 tablespoons of Ricotta cheese on each one. Lay tomato slices on top of the Ricotta.

3. Add some chicken slices on top of the tomatoes. Salt and pepper to taste. Bake at 375 for 12-15 minutes or until the Ricotta is soft and the tomatoes and chicken are heated through.

32. Spinach Sausage Egg Casserole

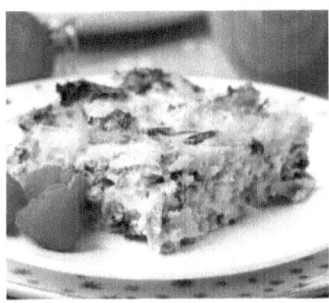

Ingredients

- 6 large eggs
- ½ cup milk or heavy cream
- 1 cup of sausage crumbles
- 1 cup of spinach, either fresh or frozen
- 1 cup shredded cheddar cheese
- 1 cup of easy biscuit mix or self-rising flour

Method

1. Preheat oven to 375 degrees. In a large bowl, whisk the eggs and milk together. Pour the eggs and milk into a greased baking dish or casserole pan.

2. Pour the sausage crumbles in with the egg mixture. Add the spinach. Add the biscuit mix and stir it throughout the pan. Pour the shredded Cheddar cheese on the top of the casserole. Bake at 375 for 20-30 minutes or until eggs are set.

33. Curry Chicken Salad

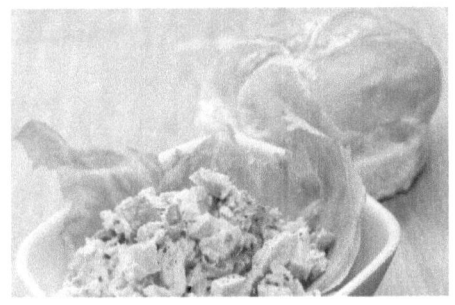

Ingredients

- 13-ounce can of chicken
- 1 yellow onion
- 1 clove of garlic
- 3 tablespoons of yellow curry powder
- ½ cup of mayonnaise
- 1 teaspoon of salt

Method

1. Dice the onion and garlic and combine them. In a large bowl mix the chicken and the onion and garlic. Use a fork so that the chicken shreds into strands. Add the curry powder and salt and mix well. Add the mayonnaise and stir well. Refrigerate for two hours before serving. Great for sandwiches and picnics.

34. Philly Cheesesteak Sandwiches

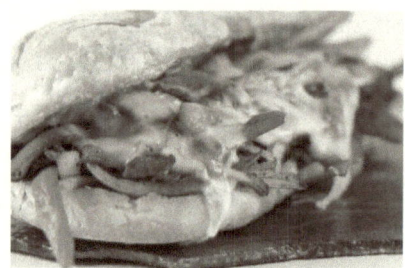

Ingredients

- 4 hoagie or sub rolls
- 1 lb. of deli roast beef sliced very thin
- ½ pound of sliced American cheese
- 1 large yellow onion
- 1 green pepper
- 4 teaspoons of olive oil
- Salt and pepper to taste

Method

1. Dice the onion. Slice the pepper into strips lengthwise. Cook the peppers and onions together in a saucepan or skillet until tender. Add the roast beef to the pan. Cook until beef is heated thoroughly and no

longer "pink" while chopping it into smaller pieces with a firm spatula. Mix well. Season with salt and pepper to taste.

2. Preheat oven to 350°F. Cut one side, lengthwise and both sides widthwise of each bun to make open-face type opening. Lay two slices of the American cheese on each side of the bun. Layer the beef and onion and pepper mixture on the buns. Close rolls shut and wrap in tin foil. Place in preheated oven on cookie sheet for 5 minutes or until heated through and cheese melts.

35. Fish Tacos

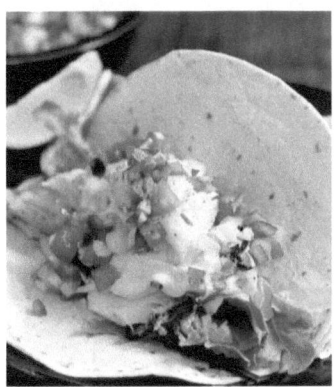

Ingredients

- Grouper
- 2 tablespoons canola oil
- 8 corn tortillas
- 1 avocado, diced
- 1 medium peach, diced
- 4 tablespoons red onion, diced
- 3/4 cup red cabbage, finely shredded
- 4 tablespoons fresh cilantro, minced
- 2 limes, quartered
- Salt and pepper to taste

Method

1. Dice the avocado, peach, onion, and cilantro. Then chop the cabbage and quarter the limes. Prepare both sides of the grouper for frying by seasoning both sides with salt and fresh ground pepper.

2. Heat oil in a large frying pan over medium-high heat. When oil is rippling, place fish in the heated pan, flesh side down. Remove the fish from the heat, and divide into 8 equal portions. (Two tacos per person)

3. Top each tortilla with a portion of the fish, and some avocado, peach, red onion, red cabbage, fresh cilantro and a generous squeeze of fresh lime juice.

36. Turkey Chili

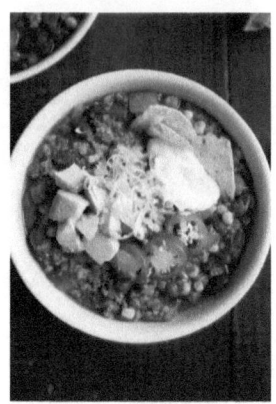

Ingredients

- 2 tablespoons olive oil
- 1 1/2 pounds ground turkey
- 3 large carrots, chopped
- 5-6 stalks celery, chopped
- 1 onion, chopped
- 4 cloves garlic, minced
- Salt and Pepper to taste
- 1 15-ounce jar tomato sauce
- 1 1/2 cups chicken stock
- 2 cups tortilla chips
- 1 cup shredded Pepper Jack cheese
- 1 16-ounce container of sour cream

Method

1. In a skillet heat the oil. Add the garlic and the onion. Cook the ground turkey in the skillet with the garlic and the onion. While that is cooking, put the carrots and celery in a pot with the chicken stock. Bring to a boil

and then simmer. Add the ground turkey mixture when the turkey is cooked.

2. Again, bring to a boil then reduce to simmer. Add the tomato sauce. Stir everything together and let it simmer for 30-60 minutes. Serve with tortilla chips and sour cream.

37. Homemade Chicken and Veggie Soup

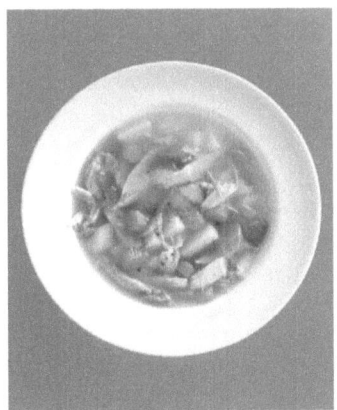

Ingredients

- 8 cups of chicken stock
- 4-ounce skinless, bone-in chicken thighs
- 12-ounce skinless, bone-in chicken breast half
- 2 cups chopped carrot
- 2 cups chopped celery
- 1 cup chopped onion
- 6 ounces uncooked medium egg noodles
- 1/2 teaspoon kosher salt
- 1/2 teaspoon black pepper

Method

1. In a large soup pot combine the chicken stock and the chicken. Bring to a boil and then simmer for 20-30 minutes or until cooked through. Remove the chicken and shred it. Return the chicken to the pot. Add the carrots, celery and onion to the pot. Bring to a boil and reduce to simmer for 10 minutes. Add the salt and pepper. Add the egg noodles and simmer until the noodles are soft.

38. Ranch Pasta Salad with Chicken

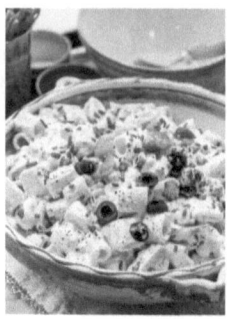

Ingredients

- 14-ounce can of chicken
- 12-ounce package of tri-color rotini pasta
- 1 cup mayonnaise or sour cream
- 1 cup of ranch salad dressing
- 1 yellow onion
- 1 clove of garlic

Method

1. Cook the pasta according to the directions on the package. Drain it well and put it I the fridge to cool. Chop the onion and the garlic. Put the chicken, onion and garlic in a bowl. Stir well.

2. In a smaller bowl, mix the mayonnaise or sour cream and the ranch dressing. Combine well. Grab the pasta from the fridge. Put it in the bowl with the chicken mixture. Stir. Stir in the mayonnaise and dressing mixture and toss to coat. Refrigerate for at least two hours before serving.

39. Sweet Potato Patties

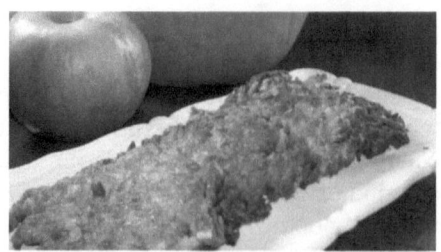

Ingredients

- 2 sweet potatoes
- 4 eggs
- 1 cup Parmesan cheese
- 1/2 teaspoon rosemary
- 1/4 teaspoon pepper
- 3 tablespoons of vegetable oil

Method

1. Preheat the oven to 425 degrees. Peel and grate the sweet potatoes into a bowl. Add the eggs. Add the Parmesan cheese, rosemary and pepper. Combine thoroughly.

2. Use a large spoon or a scoop and put a spoonful or scoopful on a greased cookie sheet. Brush olive oil on the top of each patty. Bake at 425 for 30 minutes or until golden brown and crispy. Serve with sour cream or use as a side dish.

40. Sun Dried Tomato Chicken

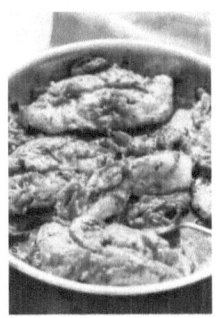

Ingredients

- 4 chicken breasts
- 2 green onions
- ¼ cup olive oil
- ¼ cup sun-dried tomatoes
- 2 tablespoons balsamic vinegar
- 1 teaspoon dried oregano
- 1 garlic clove
- Salt and pepper to taste

Method

1. Preheat the oven to 350 degrees. Chop the green onions, chop the sun-dried tomatoes and mince the garlic. In a bowl, combine the sun-dried tomatoes, balsamic vinegar, oregano, garlic, olive oil, and season with salt and pepper to taste.

2. Place the chicken breasts in a casserole or baking dish and pour the tomato mixture on top. Sprinkle the green onions over everything in the dish, and bake for 45 minutes or until the chicken is well cooked.

41. Stuffed Peppers

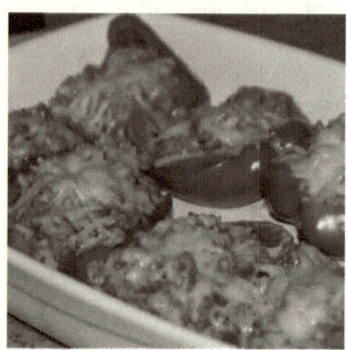

Ingredients

- 4-6 large bell peppers
- 16-ounce package of quinoa
- 1 onion
- 1 tablespoon of olive oil
- 1 clove of garlic
- 1 lb of ground turkey
- 1 zucchini
- 3 tomatoes
- 8 oz package of cream cheese cut into cubes
- 3-4 tablespoons of Italian Seasoning Mix
- Salt & pepper to taste
- 2 cups shredded Cheddar cheese

Method

1. Chop the onion, zucchini and tomatoes. Mince the garlic. Preheat the oven to 375 degrees. Cut one side off of each bell pepper and then

remove the seeds. Take the sides that you cut off and dice them then set them aside. Cook the quinoa according to the directions on the package.

2. Sauté the onion in the olive oil for 3-4 minutes on medium high heat. Add the ground turkey and the diced bell peppers to the pan. Once the ground turkey is browned add your diced zucchini and the tomatoes. Cook for about 5 minutes.

3. Add the cooked quinoa to the mixture. Add the cream cheese. Stir well until all of the cream cheese is mixed in. Add in the Italian Seasoning and the salt and pepper and mix it in well. Turn the heat off.

4. Spoon the cooked mixture into each bell pepper, making sure you fill the whole pepper. Place your stuffed peppers into a baking pan, side by side. Top them with the shredded cheese. Bake the peppers in the oven for 25-30 minutes.

42. Chicken Broccoli Pie

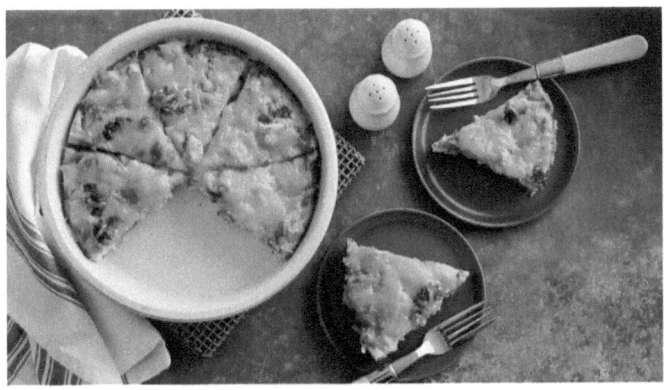

Ingredients

- 12 ounces of frozen chopped broccoli that has been thawed and drained or 12 ounces of fresh broccoli pieces
- 1 & 1/2 cups shredded Cheddar cheese
- 1 cup cut-up cooked chicken or canned chicken
- 1 medium onion, chopped
- 2 eggs
- 1 cup milk
- 1/2 cup self-rising flour or biscuit baking mix

Method

1. Preheat oven to 400 degrees. In a large bowl combine the chicken, broccoli, and 1 cup of the cheese. Spoon the chicken mixture into a 10-pie pan or a shallow baking dish.

2. In another bowl, whisk the eggs and the milk. Stir in the flour or biscuit mix. Pour that mixture into the pie pan or baking sheet. Salt and pepper to taste. Top with the rest of the shredded cheese. Bake 30-40 minutes or until a knife inserted in the center comes out clean.

43. Italian Chicken Casserole

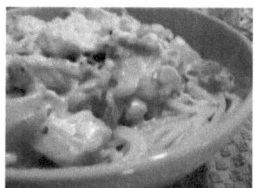

Ingredients

- 2 tablespoons of olive oil
- 1 onion, chopped
- 3 cloves of garlic, minced
- 3 cups of chicken, cooked and cubed or canned chicken
- Two 14-ounce cans of tomatoes with garlic, onion and oregano
- 1 cup of heavy whipping cream or half and half
- 6-ounce package of cream cheese, softened
- 2 cups of shredded Mozzarella cheese
- 8-ounce package of angel hair pasta

Method

1. Cook the angel hair pasta and put it aside. Keep it warm. Preheat oven to 350 degrees. In a large skillet, heat the olive oil. Add the onion and garlic. Cook until soft.

2. Add the chicken, tomatoes and heavy cream. Add the cream cheese and one cup of the Mozzarella cheese. Bring to a boil, then simmer for 10 minutes. Add the pasta. Toss everything to coat. Pour into a greased casserole dish. Top with the rest of the Mozzarella cheese and bake for 30 minutes.

44. Chicken Fried Rice

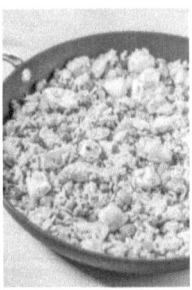

Ingredients

- 2 tablespoons of sesame oil or vegetable oil
- 1 cup cooked chicken or canned chicken, cubed
- 2 large eggs
- 1 cup carrots, sliced
- 1 cup scallions, diced
- 3 cups cooked rice
- 1 cup of frozen mixed vegetables, cooked
- ½ cup soy sauce

Method

1. This is a great way to use up leftovers. You can substitute any combination of veggies and meat that you like. Cook the rice, cook the vegetables, and cook the chicken if you need to.

2. In a skillet, heat the oil so it is sizzling. Add in the scallions, carrots, and vegetables. Cook for 2-3 minutes. Add the rice. Add the eggs. Add the soy sauce and toss everything together. Fry for 6-10 minutes.

45. Mexican Baked Potatoes

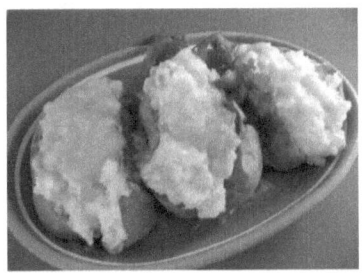

Ingredients

- 4 large russet potatoes
- 3/4 cup refried beans
- 2 scallions
- 1 package Taco seasoning
- Salt & freshly ground pepper to taste
- 3/4 cup mild or medium salsa
- 1 cup shredded cheddar cheese
- 1 cup of sour cream

Method

1. Preheat oven to 425 degrees. Wash potatoes and poke them with a fork in several places. Bake the potatoes for 40-60 minutes or until tender.

2. Slice the potato in half. Scoop out the middle of each half. Put the potato middles, refried beans, and scallions in a bowl. Add the Taco seasoning. Scoop the mixture back into the potatoes. Top with salsa and shredded Cheddar. Serve with sour cream.

46. Southwest Style Rice and Beans

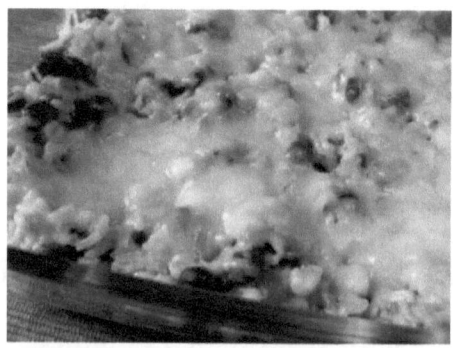

Ingredients

- 2 cups cooked white rice
- 15-ounce can of Black beans
- 15-ounce can of corn
- 1 ½ cups salsa
- Salt and Pepper to taste
- 1 ½ cups shredded Mexican or Cheddar cheese

Method

1. Preheat oven to 350 degrees. In a large bowl, combine rice, beans, corn and salsa. Pour into a greased baking dish. Salt and pepper to taste. Top with the shredded cheese. Bake for 30 minutes.

47. Chicken and Broccoli Tetrazzini

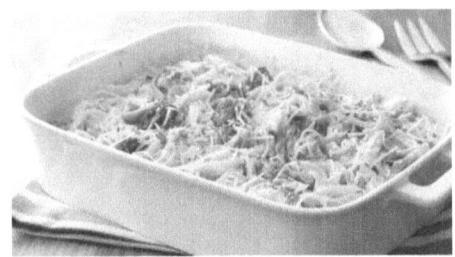

Ingredients

- 1 16-ounce package of thin spaghetti
- 1 12-ounce package frozen broccoli, cooked
- 2 cups cooked chicken
- 2 tablespoons butter
- 7 tablespoons flour
- 1 teaspoon salt
- 2 cups chicken broth
- 1 cup milk
- 1/2 cup Parmesan cheese
- 1 cup Mozzarella cheese

Method

1. Preheat the oven to 400 degrees. In a large saucepan melt the butter. Add the flour and salt and stir to combine. Cook the butter and flour mixture for 1 to 2 minutes.

2. Whisk in the chicken stock. Bring the mixture to a boil, then simmer for 2-5 minutes until it thickens. Remove from the heat and stir in the milk and Parmesan until the cheese melts.

3. Spread the broccoli and spaghetti in a greased baking dish. Top with the cooked chicken. Pour the sauce over the top. Top with the Mozzarella cheese and bake for 30 minutes.

48. Easy Taco Salad

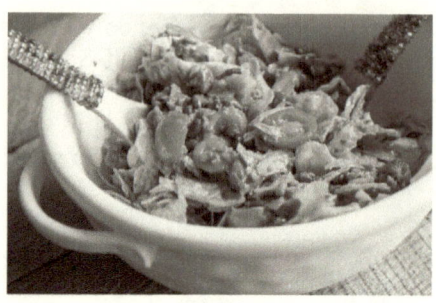

Ingredients

- pound ground beef
- 2 cups chopped yellow, red, or green bell pepper
- 2 cups salsa
- 1/4 cup chopped fresh cilantro
- 4 cups coarsely chopped romaine lettuce
- 2 cups chopped tomatoes
- 1 cup shredded cheddar cheese
- 1 cup crumbled tortilla chips
- 1/4 cup chopped green onions
- 1 cup sour cream

Method

1. Brown the ground beef in a skillet. Add the onions and peppers. Heat through. Add the salsa and cilantro. Bring to a boil.

2. Put one cup of lettuce on each plate. Pour the ground beef mixture on top of the lettuce. Add some chopped tomatoes, shredded Cheddar, and crumbled tortilla chips. Serve with sour cream on the side.

49. Stuffed Zucchini

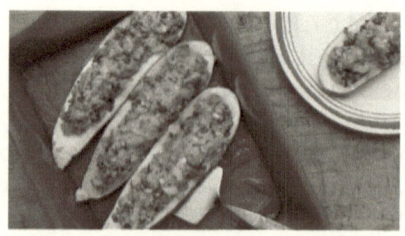

Ingredients

- 4 zucchinis
- 1 16-ounce package of pre-cooked sausage crumbles
- 1 32-ounce jar of spaghetti sauce
- 1 cup of bread crumbs
- 1 clove of garlic, minced
- 1 cup of shredded Mozzarella cheese
- 1 cup grated Parmesan cheese

Method

1. Preheat oven to 350 degrees. Slice each zucchini lengthwise. Scoop out the seeds and the insides. Put the seeds and insides in a bowl. Toss zucchini seeds with sausage crumbles, garlic, Parmesan cheese.

2. Stuff the zucchini with the sausage mixture and top with the spaghetti sauce. Cover the pan with tin foil. Cook for 45 minutes. Remove foil. Pour the Mozzarella cheese on top and bake until the cheese is melted.

50. Sausage Potatoes and Peppers

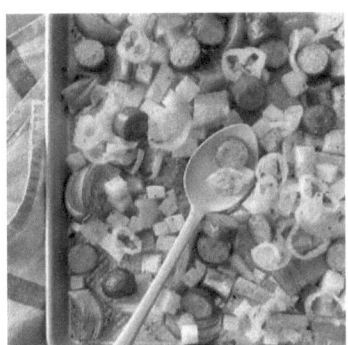

Ingredients

- 1 16-ounce package smoked sausage links
- 5 golden potatoes
- 1 jar banana peppers
- 2 bell peppers
- 1 onion
- 3 tablespoon(s) olive oil
- Salt and Pepper to taste

Method

1. Preheat oven to 400 degrees. Slice the sausage links into small discs. Wash the potatoes. Slice them into discs. Slice the onion. Slice the peppers lengthwise into long ribbons.

2. Pour the potatoes, sausage and onions into a bowl. Coat with olive oil. Salt and pepper to taste. Pour the entire bowl into a greased baking dish. Bake for 30-40 minutes or until potatoes are tender.

51. Baked Ziti

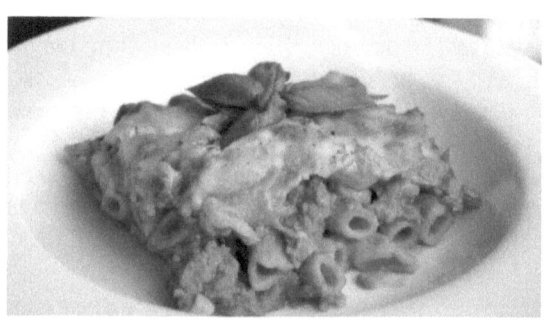

Ingredients

- 1 16-ounce package of ziti pasta
- 3 tablespoons of olive oil
- pound ground beef
- 1 large onion, chopped
- 3-4 garlic cloves, chopped
- 1 tablespoon fresh rosemary, minced
- 1 tablespoon Italian seasoning
- 1/2 teaspoon red pepper flakes
- 1 32-ounce jar of spaghetti sauce
- 1/2 pound of shredded Mozzarella cheese
- 1 cup of Ricotta cheese
- 1 cup grated Parmesan cheese

Method

1. Preheat oven to 350 degrees. Cook pasta according to the directions on package. Drain it and set aside. In a skillet, heat the olive oil. Add the onion and garlic. Cook for 3-5 minutes.

2. Add the ground beef. Cook until browned. Add the spaghetti sauce and heat through. Add the rosemary and Italian seasoning. Grease a large casserole pan or baking dish.

3. Pour some of the sauce mixture in the bottom of the dish. Layer in the pasta. Pour more of the sauce mixture on top. Layer in the ricotta cheese. Pour the rest of the sauce mixture on top. Top with the Mozzarella and Parmesan cheese. Bake for 20 minutes.

52. Green Beans in Coconut Milk

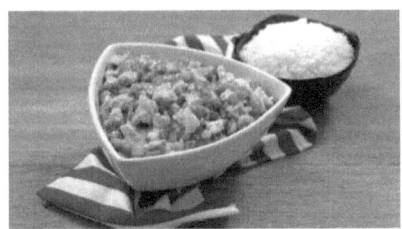

Summary

Green beans and the rich coconut milk flavor in this recipe complements well with the slight taste of chili. A good way of sharing this meal for the whole family as this not only whets the appetite but provides comforting taste and awakens the palate.

Ingredients

- 3 tablespoons of oil
- 2 cloves of garlic, chopped
- 1 small chopped onion
- 150 grams of ground pork
- 3 cups of green beans
- 1 can of coconut cream
- ½ cup of coconut milk
- 2 pieces of bird's eye chili, chopped
- Salt, pepper and sugar to taste

Method

1. Heat the oil in the pan. Sauté garlic and onions. Add the ground pork and cook thoroughly until brown. Add the green beans and coconut cream.

2. Simmer until liquid is reduced. Add coconut milk and cook until the beans are done and tender. Add chili. Season to taste. Serve hot and enjoy!

Tips

If you don't have any available fresh coconut cream and milk, powdered substitute will do for this recipe. The trick: dissolve them with the right amount of water and voila...you already have your coconut milk for this recipe.

53. Minestrone Soup with Macaroni

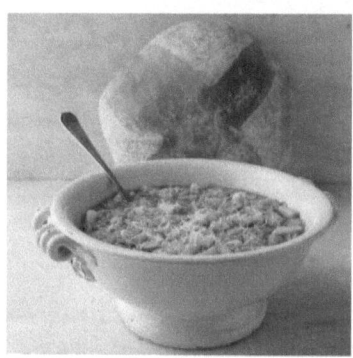

Summary

This is a complete meal in itself. It is definitely satisfying, comforting and tasty – most of all affordable and easy to prepare.

Ingredients

- 2 tablespoons of oil
- 4 cloves of minced garlic
- 1 onion (finely chopped)
- 1 red bell pepper (diced)
- 1 green bell pepper (diced)
- 1 zucchini (diced)
- ½ cup of mushroom (sliced)
- 4 cups of beef stock
- 1 cup of uncooked macaroni
- 1 can of white beans (drained)
- 1 pack of frozen mixed vegetables (small size)
- Fresh basil for garnish (chopped)

Method

1. Heat oil in a pot then sauté onions and garlic. Add red and green bell peppers, mushrooms and zucchini. Add the beef stock and bring it to a boil. Reduce heat.

2. Add macaroni pasta and cook until done. Add beans and the frozen vegetables then simmer for a few more minutes. Ladle into bowl then serve hot with chopped fresh basil on top. Enjoy!

Tips

Plain pasta, tortellini or shell pasta can also be a good substitute for this recipe.

54. Chili Beans with Pasta

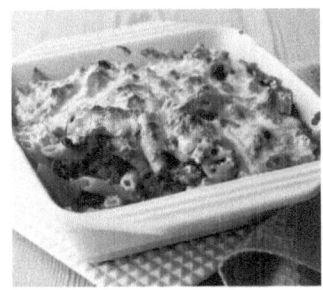

Summary

This is an easy recipe that you can prepare in just 20 minutes – a quick but delicious and nutritious meal for the whole family.

Ingredients

- 1 pound of ground beef (choose those that are lean)
- ¾ cup of onion (chopped)
- 1 15 oz. red kidney beans (drained and rinsed)
- 1 can of 14 ½ oz. diced tomatoes
- 1 can of 8 oz. tomato sauce
- ½ cup elbow macaroni (uncooked)
- 1 can of 4 oz. diced green chile peppers (drained)
- 2 teaspoons of chili powder
- ½ teaspoon of garlic salt
- ½ cup of shredded Monterey Jack (or you can use cheddar cheese)

Method

1. Cook the meat with the onions in a large skillet until brown and tender. Drain excess fat. Add the beans, diced tomatoes, macaroni, tomato sauce, chili powder, garlic salt and chile peppers. Bring to boil and then reduce heat. Cover and simmer for about 20 minutes or until your macaroni if cooked. Stir often.

2. Take out the skillet from the heat and sprinkle it with cheese. Cover and let stand for about 2 minutes. Serve and enjoy!

Tips

You can keep it kid-friendly by decreasing the amount of chili or whatever is preferred by your kids.

55. Tuna Spaghetti with Tomatoes and Garlic

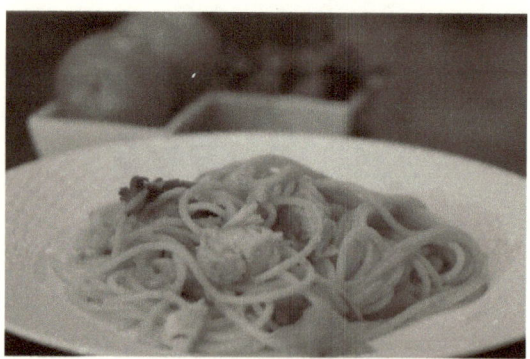

Summary

Here's another quick recipe that uses ingredients that are readily available in your pantry. Saves precious time but produces a delightful meal.

Ingredients

- 1 400-gram pack of spaghetti
- ¼ cup of olive oil
- 4 heads of garlic (chopped)
- 3-4 pieces of large, plump tomatoes (seeded and cut to strips)
- 2 cups of tuna (drained)
- Salt and pepper to taste

Method

1. Cook pasta according to label instructions. Drain and set aside. Heat your oil in the pan and sauté your garlic until it releases its aroma. Add the tomatoes and cook thoroughly.

2. Add the tuna and continue cooking until done. Add in the cooked pasta and toss them together. Add salt and pepper to taste. Serve and enjoy.

Tips

If you want to add a bit of spice in this dish, you can use the spicy kind of tuna. Tuna is rich in Omega 3 which is good for your heart.

56. Beef and Vegetable Stew

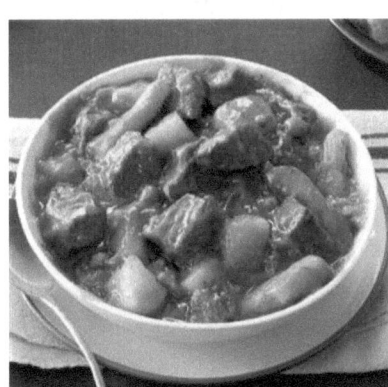

Summary

Try this protein rich and nutritious recipe that is hassle-free and budget friendly.

Ingredients

- 1 tablespoon of oil
- 2 tablespoons of garlic (chopped)
- 1 small onion (chopped)
- 500 grams of beef (cut into small cubes)
- 1 can of whole kernel corns (drained)
- 1 can of crushed tomatoes
- Salt and pepper to taste
- Spring onions (sliced to strips)

Method

1. Heat oil in a pan. Sauté onions and garlic. Add the beef and cook for a few minutes. Add the tomatoes and corn and simmer until the beef is already tender. Reduce the sauce. Season with salt and pepper then add some sliced spring onions for garnish. Serve hot and enjoy.

Tips

You can use tender cut beef so that it would cook faster. Cut them into small and uniform size so that they will be cooked evenly and all at the same time.

For some touch of herbs, you can replace the plain canned tomatoes with those that are already flavored. They are usually mixed with oregano and basil.

57. Garlic-Herb Beef Roast

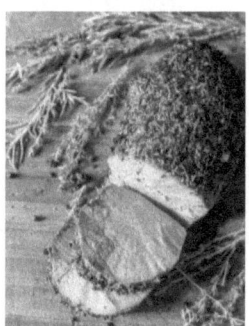

Summary

Another recipe that can be prepared in less than 30 minutes, easy to make and simple. It's a good source of protein and the addition of vegetables will provide the nutrients that your family needs.

Ingredients

- 1 oz. of beef roast au jus (refrigerated)
- 1 lb. of small red potatoes (quartered)
- 3 medium sized carrots (peeled and sliced diagonally)
- 1 tablespoon of cooking oil
- 3 tablespoons of fresh flatleaf parsley (chopped)
- 3 cloves of garlic (minced)
- 1 tablespoon of lemon peel (finely shredded)

Method

1. Cook and cover the beef roast in a large skillet over medium-high heat for about 10 minutes. Once done, simmer for another 5 minutes until its juices are reduced slightly.

2. Place the quartered potatoes and sliced carrots in a microwave safe dish. Drizzle the vegetables with oil and season with pepper. Toss slightly to even out the flavor and oil. Cover and cook inside the microwave oven on high temperature for about 10 minutes until its tender.

3. For the garlic-herb mixture, combine garlic, parsley and lemon peel in a bowl. Set aside. Stir the vegetables into the skillet with the beef roast. Place them on the serving plate and add some garlic-herb mixture. Serve hot and enjoy.

Tips

You can buy your beef roast au jus on any leading supermarkets. Add flair to this prepared meal by using this recipe instead of eating it as it is.

58. Paella in A Flash

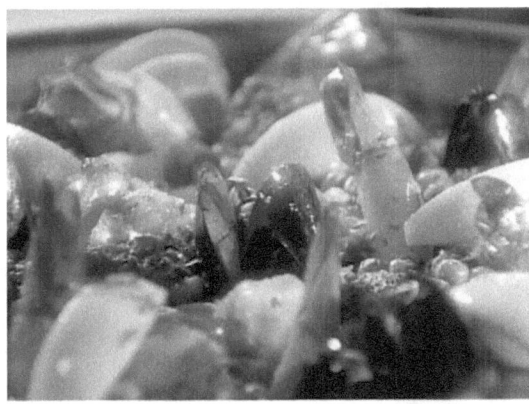

Summary

Paella is a rice dish that originated from Spain and became popular around the world. In this recipe, you will be able to prepare this dish in under 30 minutes.

This preparation is already a complete and healthy meal in itself. Ingredients are easy to find and easy to use.

Ingredients

- ¼ cup of corn oil
- 1 teaspoon of annatto powder
- 1 tablespoon of garlic (minced)
- 1 cup of onions (chopped)
- 1 small red bell pepper (sliced)
- 3 pieces of Chorizo (sliced)
- 1 cup of chicken breast (cooked and sliced into cubes)
- ¼ teaspoon of Spanish paprika
- 2 pieces of chicken bouillon cube
- 3 ½ cups of cooked rice
- Salt and pepper to taste

Method

1. In a large sauce pan, heat oil and garlic and annatto powder. Mix the onions and bell peppers. Cook until fragrant. Add in the chorizo, paprika, chicken, and the bouillon cubes. Cook until the cubes are already dissolved and incorporated in the dish.

2. Add the cooked rice and mix well. Make sure that the color will be distributed evenly on the rice. Season with salt and pepper. Serve and enjoy.

Tips

For a richer and delightful tasting paella, you can add shrimps, mussels or squid. This would also add a festive flair in your paella.

59. Baked Mushroom-Chicken Curry Rice

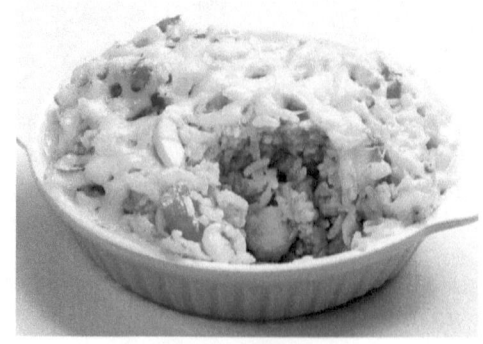

Summary

Under a tight budget? Then whip up this complete meal with your leftover ingredients and create a new and exciting dish any time.

Ingredients

- 1 can of condensed cream of mushroom soup
- ¼ cup of coconut milk
- 1/3 cup of water
- 3 tablespoons of butter
- 2 tablespoons of oil
- 3 cloves of garlic (chopped)
- 1 small onion (chopped)
- 1 chicken breast fillet (cubed)
- 6 pieces of button mushrooms (sliced)
- 2 teaspoons of curry powder
- 1 large tomato (cut to chunks)
- Salt and pepper to taste
- Mozzarella cheese (grated)

Method

1. Combine coconut milk, cream of mushroom and water in a bowl. Whisk until smooth and set aside. Heat the oil and butter together in a pan. Sauté the garlic and onions. Make sure that onions are already translucent. Cook chicken for about a minute then add the mushrooms, tomato chunks and curry powder. Mix well.

2. Add rice and combine them well to coat it evenly with the curry. Stir in the cream of mushroom mixture and mix well. Cook rice until it has a rich, creamy consistency. Add salt and pepper to taste. Transfer to an ovenproof container and top it with the mozzarella cheese. Bake in a microwave oven for 2-3 minutes on medium-high heat or until cheese melts. You can also bake it on a preheated oven with 350 degrees for about 10 minutes or until cheese melts. Serve hot and enjoy!

Tips

To save more time, you can replace your button mushrooms with canned mushrooms that are already sliced – it's fast and convenient.

60. Red Rice Soup with Beef

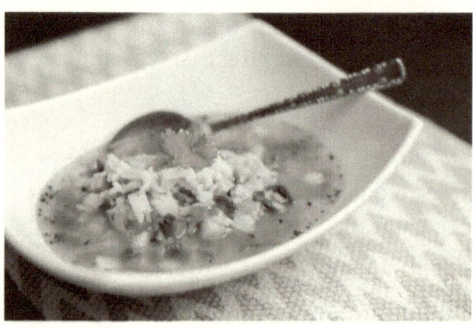

Summary

This is a simple yet nutritious comfort food that is definitely filling and heart-warming. You can make a large batch of this recipe and freeze in the refrigerator.

Simply reheat once needed and you will have an instant comfort food meal available.

Ingredients

- 1 tablespoon of canola oil
- 2.2 lbs. of beef short ribs
- 1 large white onion (chopped)
- 6 cloves of garlic (crushed and chopped)
- ½ cup of carrots (chopped)
- ½ cup of celery (chopped)
- 12 cups of water
- 1 cup of red rice (uncooked)
- Salt and pepper for tasting

Method

1. Heat oil in a very large thick-bottomed pot until hot. Sear short ribs in batches and set aside on plate. Using the same pot, sauté until translucent. Add garlic, celery, carrots and cook for a minute. Add the short ribs back in the pot and add in the water. Simmer until the ribs become soft and tender.

2. Remove the ribs. Strain the stock and remove excess fat on top of the pot. Transfer stock in another clean pot and bring to boil. Add the red

rice and the ribs. Simmer and cook around 30 minutes or until rice is thoroughly cooked. Add salt and pepper to taste. Serve and enjoy.

Tips

If you want to shorten the cook time of your ribs, you can use a pressure cooker.

61. Stir-fried Shrimp Hofan

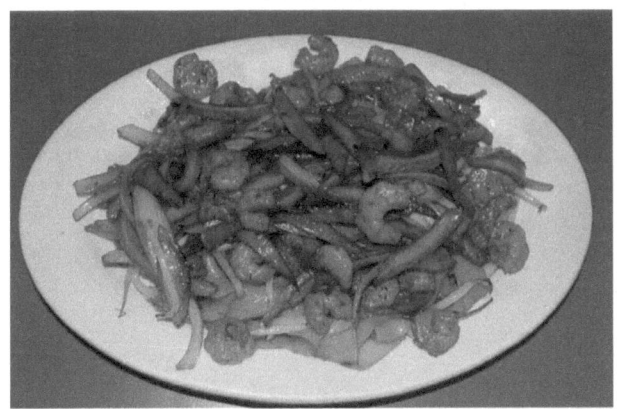

Summary

Asian cuisine is now becoming a popular choice among food lovers and consumers. In this recipe, learn to cook Asian and discover the style and its taste.

This is another way of introducing healthy, simple and a new food idea to your family.

Ingredients

- 1 pack of Hofan noodles
- 4 tablespoons of oil
- 250 grams of shrimps (shelled and deveined)
- 1 cup of bean sprouts
- 1 cake of Tofu (deep fried and sliced into thick strips)
- 1-3 tablespoons of oyster sauce
- 2 eggs (beaten)
- 2 teaspoons of water
- Salt and pepper for tasting
- ½ cups of chives (cut into thin strips)

Method

1. Cook hofan noodles as per package instructions. Drain and add 2 tablespoons of oil to avoid noodles from sticking to one another. Pour remaining oil in a pan and sauté shrimps and bean sprouts. Add in the fried tofu. Pour the beaten eggs and let it set before mixing.

2. Mix in the oyster sauce with water and pour on the pan. Add salt and pepper to taste then add the chives. Put the noodles on a serving plate and top it with the shrimp-veggie mixture. Serve hot and enjoy!

Tips

Hofan or ho fen are flat Chinese noodles. They are the same with the Italian fettuccine and also to the vermicelli noodles which are found in most Pad Thai recipes.

62. Corned Beef Hearty Soup

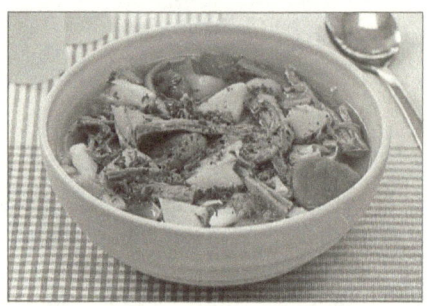

Summary

Hearty soups with soft and freshly-baked bread are perfect on any occasion. May it be for dinner or during cold seasons this recipe is proven to be filling but light on the budget.

Ingredients

- 1 tablespoon of oil
- 2 tablespoons of onions (sliced)
- 1 small can of chunky corned beef (any brand of your choice)
- 1 can of condensed cream of mushroom soup
- 1 cup of water
- 1 can of cream of corn

Method

1. Heat oil in a pot and sauté onion until translucent. Add the corned beef and cook until they are brown and a bit crusty. Add in the cream of mushroom soup, cream of corn and water. Mix thoroughly and simmer around 5 minutes. Serve hot and provide bread.

Tips

Crusty artisan breads like sourdough, multigrain loaf or ciabatta are a perfect dipping combination with this deliciously thick soup.

63. Meatloaf Pasta Parmigiana

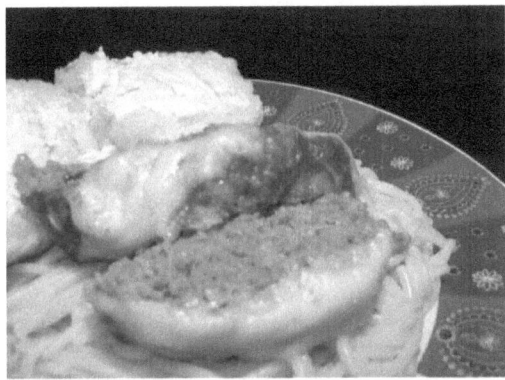

Summary

Here's a great way to use leftover meatloaf and turn it into an exciting dish for the whole family.

Ingredients

For the leftover meatloaf

- 1 cup of all-purpose flour
- 1 egg (beaten)
- 1 cup of breadcrumbs
- Oil to be used for frying
- ¼ cup of mozzarella cheese (grated)
- 1/3 cup of Parmesan cheese (grated)
- Cooked pasta

For the sauce

- 1 tablespoon of oil
- 1 tablespoon of garlic (minced)
- 1 small onion (diced)
- 1 big can of crushed tomatoes
- 1 teaspoon of dried oregano
- 1 teaspoon of dried basil
- ½ teaspoon of sugar
- Salt and pepper to taste

Method

1. Slice the leftover meatloaf then coat with flour. Dip them in beaten eggs followed by coating them on breadcrumbs. Set aside and chill for a short time. Heat the oil and cook the meatloaf until golden brown on both sides. Pat excess oil using paper towels. Set aside.

2. Heat oil then sauté onions and garlic in a saucepan. Add the tomatoes and simmer for about 10 minutes. Add more water if needed then mix in the herbs, salt and pepper. Sprinkle top of fried meatloaf with the cheeses then broil them in an oven toaster or pre-heated oven. Check to see if the cheeses are already melted then remove and set aside.

3. Toss the cooked pasta with olive oil and season with garlic powder and salt. Plate the dish with cooked pasta then topped with the sauce and meatloaf Parmigiana. Serve immediately. You can add more cheese if you want. Enjoy!

Tips

You can also use the breaded leftover meatloaf to make a healthy sandwich for your kids to take to their school.

64. Luncheon Meat Katsudon

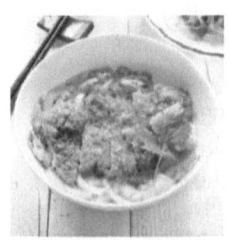

Summary

Here's another great way to use your leftover meatloaf. This time you can use another Asian flavor – let's travel in Japan. Elevate these simple canned goods into a great meal.

Ingredients

- 1 can of luncheon meat of your choice (cut them into ½ inch-thick slices)
- 1 cup all-purpose flour
- 2 eggs (beaten)
- 2 cups of Japanese bread crumbs
- Oil
- 4-6 cups of cooked rice
- 4-6 medium sized eggs
- Onion rings
- 1 medium sized carrots (julienned)
- Leeks or spring onion (chopped)

For the sauce

- 3 tablespoons of Kikkoman Soy Sauce
- ¼ cup of sugar
- Beef bouillon cube, halved (optional)
- 2 cups of water

Method

1. Slice the leftover meatloaf then coat with flour. Dip them in beaten eggs followed by coating them on breadcrumbs. Heat the oil and cook the meatloaf until golden brown on both sides.

2. Pat excess oil using paper towels. Set aside. Place all the ingredients for the sauce in a saucepan. Bring to boil and simmer for another 2 minutes.

3. Scoop a good amount of rice to individual bowls and top it with the fried meatloaf around 2- 3 slices will do. Make sure that the sauce is hot and ladle them to each of the bowl.

4. Break an egg on top of each bowl with the sauce and garnish with carrots, onion ring and spring onions. Serve and enjoy!

Tips

In making Katsudon, make sure that your sauce is piping hot to make sure that the eggs will be completely cooked on its own heat.

65. Seafood Fried Rice

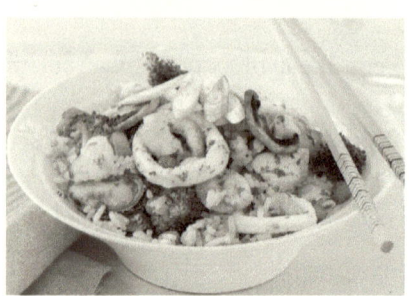

Summary

Try this complete meal in a flash. Increase your fiber and vitamin B intake with this delicious and convenient meal. Another Asian inspired meal that will surely satisfy your hungry family members.

Ingredients

- 2 tablespoons of canola oil (or peanut oil)
- 1 tablespoon of garlic (chopped)
- 2 tablespoons of onions (chopped)
- 2 tablespoons of spring onions (chopped)
- 1 Chinese sausage (cubed finely)
- 3 eggs (beaten)
- 12 cups of brown rice (cooked)
- ½ cup of shrimps
- ½ cup of clam meat
- ¼ cup of dried squid flakes (shredded)
- 3 tablespoons of soy sauce
- 1 teaspoon of sweet-chili sauce

Method

1. Heat oil in a large wok and sauté onions, garlic and spring onions until you can smell the fragrance. Combine the sausage with the beaten egg. Mix well until the eggs are thoroughly cooked.

2. Add the other ingredients and stir-fry until shrimps change color and get cooked. Make sure that all of the ingredients are evenly combined with the rice. Serve hot and enjoy!

Tips

The secret to making an awesome fried rice is to make sure that all ingredients are mixed and combined well. So better get ready to stir, stir, stir!

66. Cajun Pork Chops with Gravy

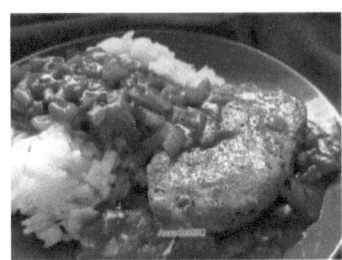

Summary

This is a proven family favorite in every home. Who can resist the tasty Cajun flavors topped with gravy? Come on and give it a try!

Ingredients

- 6 pieces of pork chops (choose the lean ones)
- 1 cup of onion (chopped)
- 1 cup of green pepper (chopped)
- 1 cup of celery (chopped)
- 1 cloves of garlic (crushed)
- 1 pack of beef gravy (prepared per package instructions)
- 3 cups of rice (cooked)
- Vegetable oil
- Cajun seasoning
- Salt and pepper to taste

Method

1. Rub the chops with Cajun seasonings liberally. Place a small amount of oil in the pan. Sear the chops and both sides then set aside. Put the onion, celery, garlic and pepper to the pan and sauté until fragrant.

2. Add the pork chops back into the pan and pour in the prepared gravy on it. Simmer for about 45 minutes. Serve hot over cooked rice and enjoy!

Tips

Cajun seasoning mostly consists of a blend of salt and variety of spices such as cayenne pepper and garlic.

67. Chicken Barbecue with Java Rice

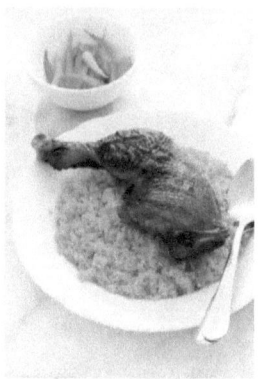

Summary

Tried and tested recipe that would bring satisfaction to your whole family. Every bite has a taste of sweet, tangy and juicy fillets combined with the perfect blend of java rice.

Ingredients

- 4 pieces of chicken breast fillet
- ½ cup of store bought barbecue marinade

For the Java Rice

- 3 tablespoons of annatto oil
- 1 teaspoon of garlic (minced)
- ¾ cup ground pork
- 4 cups of rice (cooked)
- Salt and pepper to taste
- Peanut sauce for dipping (optional)

Method

1. Combine chicken and barbecue marinade in a bowl for 2-4 hours. Place them on the refrigerator. Heat grill or you may use a grill pan, until it is very hot. Put the marinated chicken on the pan and cook for about 2-3 minutes on both sides. Make sure to lower the heat to avoid burning the chicken. Set aside.

2. In making the java rice: In the pan, heat the annatto oil. Sauté garlic and add the ground until cooked. Add the cooked rice and mix them well. Add salt and pepper to taste. Remove from the heat and set aside. Transfer the rice to a serving plate then place the barbecued chicken with the peanut sauce. Serve hot and enjoy!

Tips

Try marinating your chicken meat for 24 hours. This would allow more time for the marinade mix to be fully incorporated in the meat making it much tastier.

68. Egg and Spinach Sandwiches

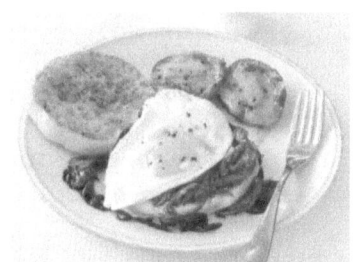

Summary

Thought that eggs are only good for breakfast? Guess again. Try out this recipe and it will surely make you want for more. Fast, delicious and healthy. It might make your kids eat vegetables too.

Ingredients

- 4 pieces of tomatoes (halved lengthwise)
- 4 pieces of English muffins (split)
- 2 ½ tablespoons of extra virgin olive oil
- ¼ red onion (thinly sliced)
- ¼ lbs. Canadian Bacon sliced (cut into thin strips)
- 8 cups of baby spinach

- 4 large eggs
- 1/3 cup of cheddar cheese
- Salt and pepper to taste

Method

1. Preheat your broiler. Arrange the tomatoes with the cut side up on a baking tray. Season them with salt and pepper. Broil them until they are soft for about 2 minutes. Remove it from the broiler. Place the English muffins on the baking tray and brush it with a tablespoon of olive oil then set aside. Heat another tablespoon of olive oil in a nonstick pan over medium-high heat. Cook the onion until translucent around 2 minutes. Cook then the sliced Canadian bacon until slightly browned and add in the spinach until it turns wilted. Add salt and pepper to taste then transfer to them in a bowl and keep them warm.

2. Add the remaining ½ tablespoon of olive oil on the pan and cook the eggs sunny side up in the pan. Add salt and pepper to taste. Place the cheese on top of the tomatoes. Return them with the English muffin on the broiler and let the cheese melt. Separate the muffins on each plate and top it with the tomato, spinach and bacon mixture and add the fried egg. Place on top with broiled tomatoes. Serve and enjoy!

Tips

You can replace spinach with either kale, chard or collard greens. These veggies are also packed with the nutrients your body needs.

69. Roast Chicken with Potatoes and Butternut Squash

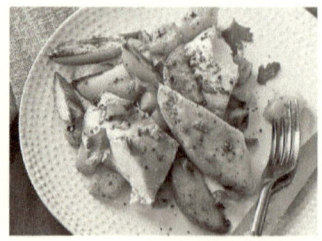

Summary

Catering just the right amount of protein combined with carbohydrates, fibers and nutrients, this nutritious dish will keep you full for a long time and that too, by spending just $1.62 per serving!

Ingredients

- 3 ½ lbs. roasting chicken
- 8 oz. cubed butternut squash
- 2 tablespoons minced garlic
- 12 oz. red potatoes, cut into wedges
- 2 tablespoons butter
- ½ teaspoon dried sage
- 1 teaspoon salt
- 3/4th teaspoon ground black pepper
- Cooking spray

Method

1. Combine dried sage, ½ teaspoon of salt, ½ teaspoon of black pepper and 1 ½ tablespoons of garlic in a small bowl. Rub the prepared garlic mixture under the skin of chicken. Place the chicken on a greased rack of broiler pan.

2. Arrange the vegetables around the chicken, season with salt and black pepper and broil in a 400 degrees Fahrenheit preheated oven for 1 hour. Let the chicken stand at room temperature for 10 minutes. Discard skin, slice and serve with vegetables.

Tips

Pair dry Riesling wine, which has a sweet peachy and orangey aroma with this dish for the perfect yet affordable drink to complement the dish.

70. Chicken and Rice with Broccoli

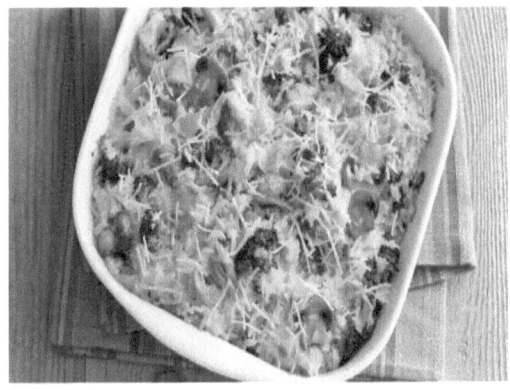

Summary

A complete meal in itself and loaded with all the necessary nutrients, this comforting dish is fabulous for freezing as well. Perfect for parties, you can be rest assured to garner some accolades for your cooking skills with this dish.

Ingredients

- 2 ½ lbs. chicken legs, bone-in and skin-on
- 3 cups chicken broth, low-sodium
- 2 cups fresh broccoli florets
- 3 garlic cloves, peeled and minced
- 1 ½ cups chopped onion
- 1 ½ cups long-grain rice
- 2 tablespoons fresh parsley, chopped
- 2 tablespoons olive oil
- 1 teaspoon of saffron threads
- Ground black pepper
- Kosher salt, to taste
- 1/4th teaspoon cayenne pepper

Method

1. Season chicken with salt and black pepper. Cook the chicken legs skin-side down in a hot greased skillet for 6-7 minutes. Flip chicken pieces and brown the other side for an additional 5 minutes. Set aside.

2. Soften the onions and broccoli florets with a pinch of salt for 2-3 minutes. Add cayenne, garlic and saffron threads. Cook for an additional 30 seconds. Pour chicken broth into the pan. Spread rice in the pan and place chicken pieces on top. Cover and cook for 15-20 minutes. Sprinkle chopped parsley on top to serve.

Tips

To retain the crunchiness of the broccoli florets, add those at the end of the cooking.

71. Chipotle Chicken Casserole

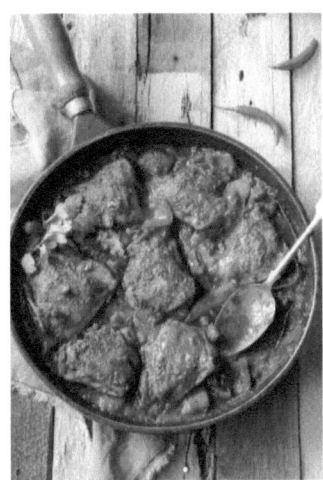

Summary

Easy to make and super healthy, your kids will simply love this casserole. It is also ideal for carrying to picnics or for serving to guests, as you will be able to serve this fancy dish at a pretty affordable rate.

Ingredients

- 1 lb. chicken breast halves, boneless
- 2 cups corn kernels, fresh or frozen
- 2 chipotle peppers in adobo sauce, roughly chopped
- 3 cups frozen hash brown potatoes, chopped
- 1/4th teaspoon chili powder
- 3/4th cup shredded Monterey Jack cheese
- 1 tablespoon olive oil
- 14 ½ oz. diced tomatoes with oregano, garlic and basil
- ½ teaspoon dried oregano
- 1/4th teaspoon ground cumin
- 1/4h teaspoon salt
- ½ teaspoon chili powder

Method

1. Brown the corns lightly in a greased skillet for 5 minutes. Add potatoes and cook for an additional 5-8 minutes. Add-in the chipotle peppers, tomatoes, ½ teaspoon of ground cumin, ½ teaspoon of chili powder and oregano. Transfer mixture to a greased 2-quarts round casserole dish.

2. Sprinkle salt, cumin and 1/4th teaspoon of chili powder over the chicken pieces. Brown chicken in the same skillet for 3-4 minutes per side. Transfer chicken breasts to the casserole dish. Bake in a 375 degrees Fahrenheit preheated oven for 20-22 minutes. Sprinkle shredded cheese after removing casserole from oven and serve warm.

Tips

You can easily pack the dish for your journey. For that, simply wrap up the casserole in aluminum foil and then wrap the packet in a heavy towel. Pack the entire packaging into an insulated container to keep it warm.

72. Turkey Sausage Mushroom and Potato Gratin

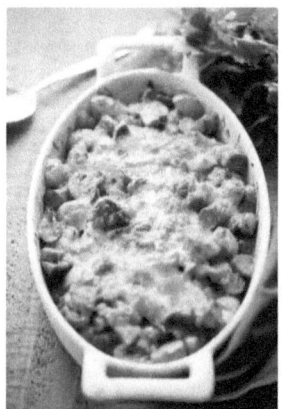

Summary

Treat your hunger with this extremely comforting dish. This dish is superbly easy to prepare and is perfect for dinner or brunch.

Ingredients

- 8 oz. hot Italian turkey sausage links, casing-removed
- ½ cup chicken broth
- 1 tablespoon butter
- 4 oz. sliced cremini mushrooms
- 3 oz. shredded Swiss cheese
- 3 cups chopped onions
- 1 ½ lbs. red potatoes, chopped
- ½ teaspoon kosher salt

Method

1. Sauté and crumble sausage links in a greased skillet over medium-high heat for 5 minutes. Remove from pan once cooked. Clean the skillet with paper towels and melt the butter in it. Throw the onions in the skillet and cook for 4 minutes. Add the mushrooms after 4 minutes and cook for 6 more minutes.

2. Add potatoes and sauté the mixture for an additional 5 minutes. Stir-in the chicken broth and the cooked sausage. Spoon-out the mixture in a greased baking dish. Sprinkle cheese on top and bake covered with an aluminum foil in a 400 degrees Fahrenheit preheated oven for 30 minutes. Remove the foil and bake for an extended 15 minutes.

Tips

To speed up the process of cooking, use ground hot turkey instead of turkey sausage links.

73. Chicken Focaccia Sandwich Recipe

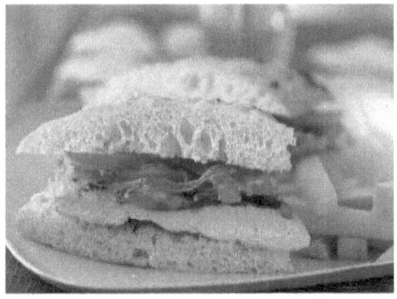

Summary

Prepare it fresh for an outing or make it ahead of time, this delicious chicken focaccia sandwich is absolutely customizable and gets prepared in a jiffy.

Ingredients

- 2 cups deli-roasted shredded or sliced chicken
- 1 large Italian focaccia bread
- 3.5 oz. roasted sweet peppers, cut into strips
- 1/3rd cup low-fat salad dressing
- 1 cup fresh basil

Method

1. Slice the bread in half. Spread salad dressing on the cut-side of the bread halves. Place basil leaves between bread halves. Top those off with chicken and sweet pepper slices. Cut the sandwich in quarters and serve.

Tips

Use onion or tomato flavored focaccia bread or you can even use sourdough bread to experience intense flavors.

74. Ginger Turkey Stir Fry

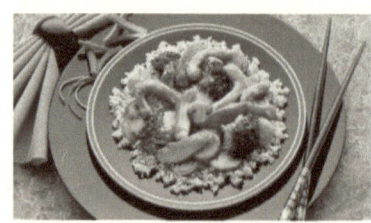

Summary

A highly nutritious meal, which is also versatile in itself, this dish can be prepared by using simple leftover foods from your fridge.

Ingredients

- 1 lb. turkey breast slices, skinless and boneless
- 2 cups sliced mushrooms
- 3 tablespoons of reduced-sodium soy sauce
- 1 cup brown rice
- 1 head napa cabbage, shredded
- 4 garlic cloves, chopped
- 2 tablespoons olive oil
- 4 teaspoons sesame seeds
- 2 cups pea pods
- 4 garlic cloves, peeled and finely chopped
- 4 green onion stalks, greens and bulbs chopped
- 1 tablespoon grated ginger
- 2 tablespoons sesame oil
- 1 teaspoon ground black pepper

Method

1. Cook the brown rice according to packaging directions. Cook turkey strips in a skillet that has been greased with olive oil for 3-4 minutes. Add to the turkey, the cabbage, ginger, peas, green onions, garlic and mushroom slices. Season the mixture with black pepper. Toss rice with sesame oil and soy sauce. Serve rice in bowls. Top with turkey stir-fry mixture and sesame seeds.

Tips

Make sure that you cook the rice by following the exact cooking directions as provided in its packaging. This will ensure that you get perfectly cooked rice.

75. Potato Crusted Chicken Fingers

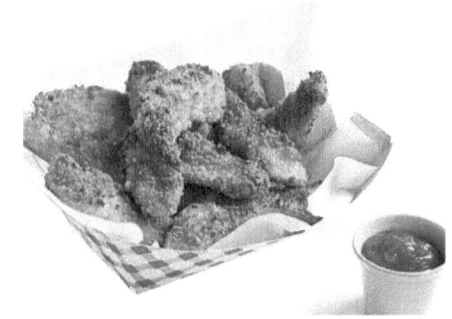

Summary

If you are a fan of chicken fingers and have failed miserably trying to get the crunchiest and juiciest chicken fingers at your home, you should definitely try this recipe. Serve a small army under just $10 and see people adding brownie points to your cooking skills.

Ingredients

- 6 oz. halved chicken breasts, skinless and boneless
- 3/4th cups all-purpose flour
- 3 eggs, lightly beaten
- 6 oz. baked potato chips
- ½ cup reduced-fat 2% milk
- 3 tablespoons canola oil
- ½ teaspoon salt

Method

1. Grind the potato chips roughly, without turning those into a powder. Transfer to a shallow dish. Season chicken breasts with salt and dredge those in flour. Combine the eggs and milk in a bowl and set aside. Transfer the flour-dipped chicken pieces to the milk mixture and then finally coat with ground potato chips.

2. Cook half of the coated chicken breasts in 1 ½ tablespoons of canola oil in a skillet for 2 minutes on each side over medium-high heat. Cook the remaining chicken in the same manner. Serve with ketchup or broccoli.

Tips

Instead of grinding the potato chips in a food processor, use a mortar and pestle for the purpose. This will crush the chips without transforming those into a powder.

76. Ham Casserole

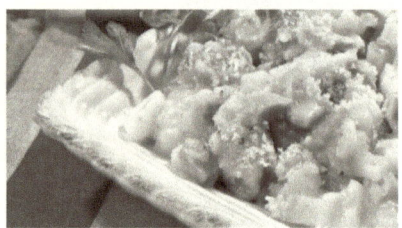

Summary

Made of just a few easily-available ingredients, this hearty ham casserole can be prepared under just $5 for an entire family.

Ingredients

- 2 cups diced ham
- 1 cup milk
- 2 cups sharp cheddar cheese, shredded
- 2 cups cooked white or brown rice
- 1 package frozen peas
- Breadcrumbs
- 1 can of cream mushroom soup

Method

1. Preheat oven to 350 degrees Fahrenheit and grease a casserole dish with cooking spray. Spread the rice in the casserole dish and layer ham and peas over the rice.

2. Combine cheese, milk and cream of mushroom soup in a bowl and pour the mixture over the rice. Finally, sprinkle breadcrumbs on top and bake for 45 minutes or until the casserole turns bubbly and its top is browned.

Tips

If you are using frozen peas, you can reduce the cooking time of the recipe by as much as 5 minutes by simply thawing the peas beforehand or by putting those in the microwave for a minute.

77. Shredded Pork Tacos

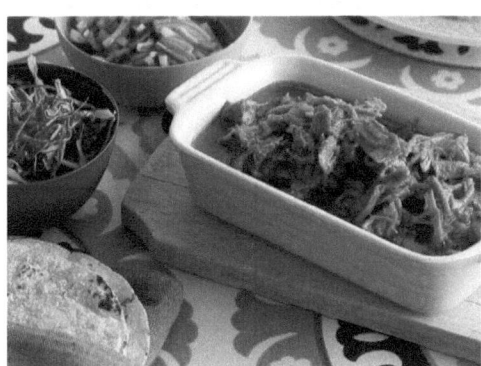

Summary

You must have your own secret recipe for making shredded pork. However; you can get a little daring here and try out this awesome recipe to pacify your hunger for delicious food.

Ingredients

- 3 lbs. pork roast
- 4 soft taco shells or tortillas
- Sour cream
- 1 cup chicken broth
- ½ cup enchilada sauce

Method

1. Cook the pork roast in a slow cooker with chicken for 8-10 hours on low or for 4-5 hours on high setting. Shred the meat once it's cooked. Reserve 2 cups of pork and set aside the rest for future use. Cook the pork for 10 minutes over medium-low heat with enchilada sauce in a saucepan.

2. Heat up the tortillas on a girdle in the meantime. Spoon the pork mixture in tortillas and serve the tacos with avocado, lettuce, cheese blend or slice olives.

Tips

If you want to add a crunch to the tacos, you can better opt for hard taco shells instead of soft shells or flour tortillas.

78. Maple Chili Gazed Pork Medallions

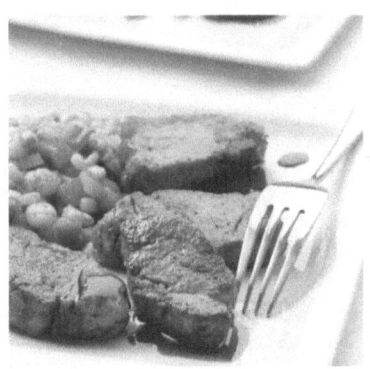

Summary

Can be prepared within just 10 minutes, this pork recipe is so delicious that you will remember its taste for years and, what's good, you will be able to prepare it right at your home without spending a penny more than $10!

Ingredients

- 1 lb. pork tenderloins, cut into 1-inch thick medallions
- 1 teaspoon chili powder
- 1 tablespoon maple syrup
- 1/4th cup apple cider vinegar
- 2 teaspoons canola oil

- ½ teaspoon salt
- 1/8th teaspoon ground chipotle

Method

1. Sprinkle chipotle pepper, salt and chili powder on both sides of pork medallions. Cook the pork medallions in canola oil in a skillet for 1-2 minutes on each side. Add apple cider vinegar and maple syrup. Bring the sauce to a boil.

2. Once the sauce starts boiling, turn down the heat to medium and cook for 1-2 minutes more. Serve the pork medallions in serving plates and drizzle the sauce on top.

Tips

Make shallow slits in the pork medallions to allow those to cook faster and to allow the meat to absorb the flavors better.

79. Maple Brined Pork

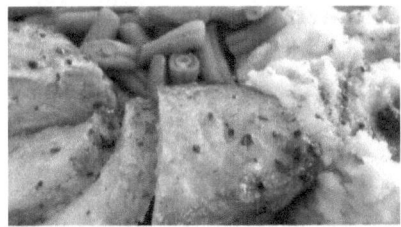

Summary

The perfect dinner recipe for a get-together, this gorgeous dish will let you experience the best of flavors you can impart to pork and that too within your budget!

Ingredients

- 4 oz. pork chops, boneless
- 2 ripe plums, pitted and halved
- 4 whole garlic cloves, peeled and crushed
- 2 tablespoons melted butter
- 1 bay leaf
- 1 ½ teaspoons allspice
- ½ cup low-sodium chicken broth

- 2 ½ tablespoons maple syrup
- 3 cups water
- 1 teaspoon black peppercorns
- 2 ripe peaches, pitted and halved
- ½ teaspoon black pepper
- 2 ½ tablespoons kosher salt

Method

1. Pour water and chicken broth in a pan and to that, add the bay leaf, allspice, garlic, 2 tablespoons of salt, peppercorns and 2 tablespoons of salt. Bring the sauce to a boil. Once done, transfer the cooled sauce and pork chops to a freezer-compatible zip-lock pouch. Chill the pork in refrigerator for 8 hours.

2. Once the time elapses, drain the sauce from pouch and retain the pork chops. Sprinkle remaining salt and black pepper over the pork chops. Grill the pork chops on a preheated greased grill for 3 minutes on each side.

3. Combine butter and ½ teaspoon of maple syrup. Brush the mixture over the pork tenderloins and sprinkle 1/4th teaspoon of ground pepper and salt. Grill the peach and plums cut-side down for 3 minutes. Serve pork with grilled fruits.

Tips

To make juicier brined pork, inject some of the brine solution into the pork tenderloins before cooking.

80. Slow Cooker Pulled Pork

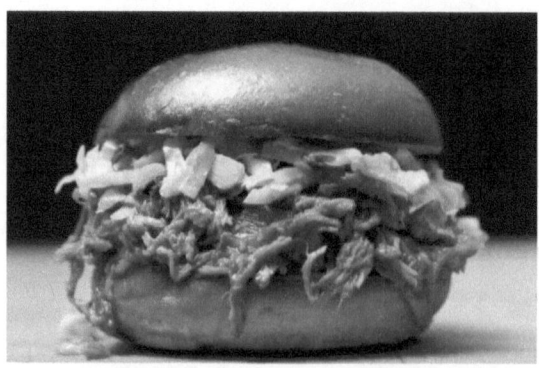

Summary

A fabulously easy recipe that calls for just 3 ingredients, you will want to cook this recipe every day for your family and even for serving to your guests, as its super-easy on pocket as well.

Ingredients

- 3 lbs. pork roast
- 18 oz. barbecue sauce
- 1 packet onion soup mix

Method

1. Place the pork roast in slow cooker. Pour onion soup mix and half the amount of barbecue sauce over the meat. Cook the pork on low for 8-9 hours or on high for 5-6 hours. Shred the cooked pork and serve between buns.

Tips

Make the barbecue sauce ahead of time at your home, so that you can simply throw everything into your slow cooker and let it do the cooking while you relax!

81. Cornmeal Crusted Pork

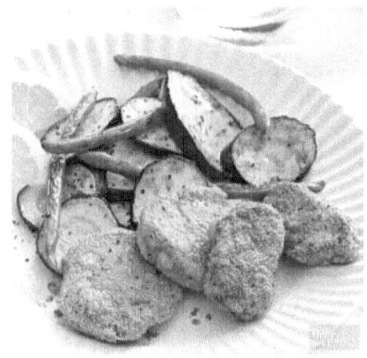

Summary

A quick, light and healthy dinner recipe, which you will want to cook on almost a regular basis, this crusted pork recipe is super easy to prepare and even easier to make it disappear within minutes of serving it.

Ingredients

- 1 lb. pork tenderloin, cut into ½-inch thick pieces
- ½ cup cornmeal
- 12 oz. green beans
- 1 egg, lightly beaten
- 2 tablespoons fresh oregano leaves
- 1 tablespoon water
- 2 zucchinis, thinly sliced
- ½ teaspoon salt
- 2 tablespoons olive oil
- ½ teaspoon black pepper

Method

1. Combine egg and water in a bowl. Dip the pork pieces in eggs mixture and then coat with cornmeal. Cook the pork pieces over medium-high heat in oil for 2 minutes on each side. Once done, set aside on a paper towel-lined plate. Cook the zucchini and beans for 6-8 minutes in the same pan. Toss with salt and pepper once cooked. Serve pork alongside zucchini and beans.

Tips

To hasten the process of cooking the vegetables, add salt while cooking. This will render the vegetables soft by taking out water from them.

82. Grilled Pork with Pineapple

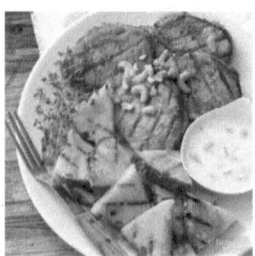

Summary

Made up of just 4-5 ingredients which are readily available in our kitchens almost regularly, this delicious pork recipe along with the orange marmalade-yoghurt dip can be prepared all within your budget.

Ingredients

- 4 boneless pork chops
- 1 fresh pineapple (peeled, cored and sliced)
- 1/4th cup roasted salted cashew, chopped
- 3 tablespoons orange marmalade
- Salt
- ½ cup yoghurt
- Ground black pepper

Method

1. Season pork with salt and pepper. Grill the pork chops and pineapple slices over medium heat for 4 minutes. Flip meat and pineapple pieces. Brush those with 2 tablespoons of orange marmalade. Grill chops and fruits for 3-5 minutes more. Combine remaining marmalade with yoghurt. Serve the pork chops and pineapple slices with yoghurt mixture, topped with chopped nuts.

Tips

Pork chops can get cooked fast. Hence, if you want to cook your pork chops perfectly, you should take the internal temperature of the pork with a meat thermometer, which should register 160 degrees Fahrenheit.

83. Crockpot Chili

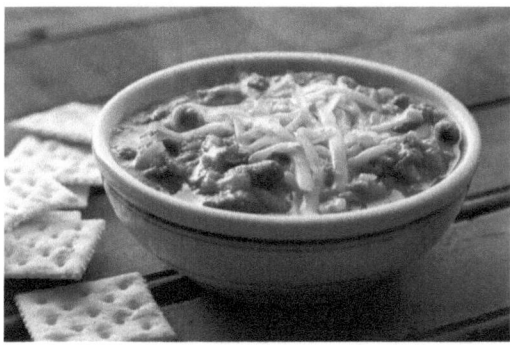

Summary

Serve your family a bowl of this heartwarming and comforting chili, without compromising with your favorite ingredients or your budget.

Ingredients

- 1 lb. lean ground beef
- 12 oz. tomato sauce
- 15 oz. kidney beans
- 2 ripe tomatoes, diced
- 1 package chili seasoning
- 1/8th red onion, diced

Method

1. Brown the beef. Drain excess fat from pan and stir-in the chili seasoning, kidney beans and tomato sauce. Dump mixture into crock pot. Add onions and tomatoes. Cook chili on low for 4-6 hours. Serve with tortilla chips or sour cream or cheddar cheese.

Tips

The trick to cooking chili the fastest way is to precook the beef and to cook the chili the next day in slow cooker. Simply cook, pack and freeze the beef, the day prior to cooking the chili.

84. Classic Meatloaf

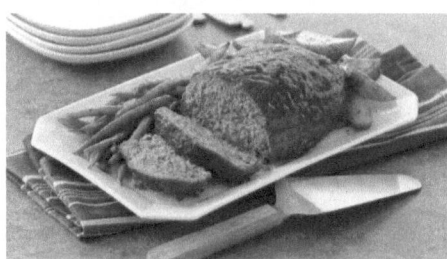

Summary

What can be better than to treat your taste buds with the comforting taste of meatloaf and that too without spending more than $10 to feed your entire family? Make sure you try your hands at this meatloaf.

Ingredients

- 1 lb. ground sirloin
- 2 teaspoons minced garlic
- 1 egg

- 1/3rd cup chopped green onions
- ½ teaspoon dry mustard
- 6 tablespoons ketchup
- 1/4th teaspoon crushed red pepper
- 1/8th teaspoon salt
- 3 tablespoons breadcrumbs
- 1/4th teaspoon black pepper

Method

1. Combine all ingredients, except for 2 tablespoons of ketchup with meat. Transfer meat to a greased loaf pan and shape accordingly. Bake meatloaf in a 400 degrees Fahrenheit oven for 20 minutes. Brush the top of meatloaf with remaining ketchup and bake for an additional 7 minutes. Slice and serve.

Tips

This meatloaf can be turned into a gluten-free meatloaf by simply using crushed oats instead of breadcrumbs.

85. Asian Beef Steak Noodles

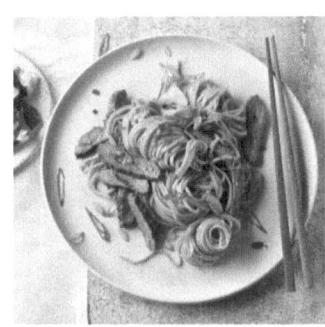

Summary

Ideal for hot summer days, this Asian beef steak noodles is not only easy to cook but is also heart and liver-healthy. It will cost you just $7-8 to serve an entire family of 4.

Ingredients

- 8 oz. beef steak, cut into ½-inch thick cubes
- 4 tablespoons sliced water chestnuts

- ½ small red bell pepper, sliced
- 3 tablespoons hoisin sauce
- 5 roasted and salted peanuts, chopped
- 7 oz. cooked noodles
- 1 tablespoon red wine vinegar
- 1/4th cup water
- 2 tablespoons vegetable oil

Method

1. Stir-fry bell pepper and water chestnut for 1 minute over medium-high heat. Combine water, vinegar and hoisin sauce. Stir-in cooked noodles and ½ of hoisin sauce mixture with the bell peppers. Transfer mixture to a bowl.

2. Cook the beef steaks with remaining hoisin sauce in the same skillet over medium-high heat for 2 minutes. Serve noodles with steaks and sprinkle chopped peanuts on top.

Tips

To add a little crunch to the recipe, you can add cucumbers to the noodles.

86. Sloppy Joe Bake

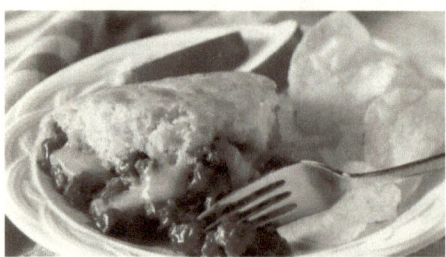

Summary

Why restrict treating your taste buds with sloppy Joe, when you can opt for this super-easy, delicious and healthy sloppy Joe bake within your budget?

Ingredients

- 1 ½ lbs. ground beef
- 3 cups cooked rotini pasta
- 1 cup shredded cheddar cheese

- 1 ½ cups chopped yellow onion
- ½ cup water
- 15.5 oz. sloppy Joe sauce

Method

1. Brown beef and onion in a skillet. Set aside in a greased baking dish. Mix sloppy Joe sauce, pasta and water with the beef mixture. Cover with aluminum foil and bake beef in a 350 degrees Fahrenheit preheated oven for 35-40 minutes. Remove cover after 40 minutes, sprinkle cheese on top and bake for an additional 5 minutes. Let stand for 5 minutes and serve.

Tips

To add an intense flavor to the sloppy Joe bake, try to brown the onions prior to browning the beef.

87. Quick Beef Stir Fry

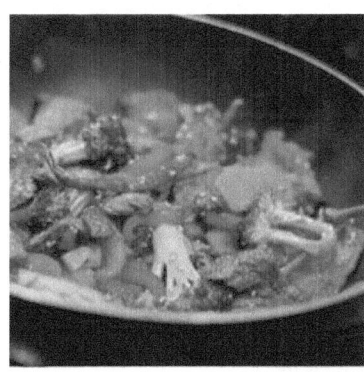

Summary

Beef stir fry is one dinner/lunch option that you can make within just a few minutes and this recipe will let you customize itself completely according to your budget.

Ingredients

- 1 lb. beef sirloin, cut into strips
- 1 teaspoon minced garlic
- 1 red bell pepper, sliced
- 1 tablespoon soy sauce

- 1 ½ cups broccoli florets
- 2 tablespoons sesame seeds
- 1 green onion, chopped
- A pinch of red pepper flakes
- 2 tablespoons vegetable oil

Method

1. Brown beef in a skillet with vegetable oil. Set aside. Stir-fry the vegetables in same skillet and add pepper flakes, soy sauce and garlic. Mix beef with vegetables. Stir-fry for 2-3 minutes and serve by sprinkling sesame seeds on top.

Tips

Customize the recipe as per your convenience and taste by adding a bit of salt and flavorings or by altering the vegetables with any vegetables of your liking.

88. Classic Pastie Slab

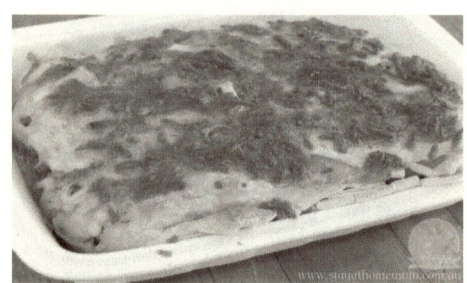

Summary

This crumbly yet juicy pasty slab is easy to put together and you can even involve your kids in the process. This makes a perfect budget-meal for a get-together dinner party.

Ingredients

- 2 carrots, cubed
- 1.1 oz. minced beef sausage
- 2 puff pastry sheets
- 2 potatoes, peeled and cubed
- 1 cup thinly sliced cabbage
- 1 egg

- 1 onion, diced
- Salt
- 1 cup grated cheese
- Black pepper

Method

1. Steam the vegetables in a pan until tender. Stir-in cheese, salt and pepper. Brown sausage separately and then mix with vegetables mixture. Line a greased baking tray with 1 pastry sheet. Spoon out meat mixture over the puff pastry.

2. Top with another puff pastry, brush the top with beaten egg and fold the pastry at the sides to form an envelope. Bake in a medium heated oven until the top of the pastry is lightly browned. Serve!

Tips

You can use other vegetables like zucchini, pumpkin and even broccoli to make the dish healthier and tastier.

89. Picadillo

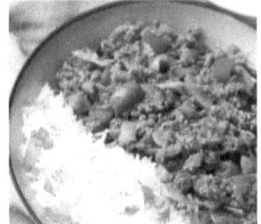

Summary

Though nothing fancy, you can be rest assured that your kids as well as any guests you are serving will definitely like this recipe. It's not only super tasty but minimal usage of oil also ensures its high health-quotient.

Ingredients

- 1 lb. lean hamburger meat
- 18 oz. tomato sauce
- 1 white onion, diced

- 1 bay leaf
- 3 garlic cloves, minced
- Salt
- 2 carrots, diced
- 2-3 chipotle peppers in adobo sauce
- 2 potatoes, diced
- Pepper

Method

1. Sauté onion, garlic and carrots in a large pan, until aromatic. Stir-in the meat and brown that while trying to crumble it. Blend the chipotle peppers and tomato sauce in a blender. Set aside.

2. Add the potatoes and bay leaf to the meat mixture. Cook for another 4-5 minutes. Add the tomato sauce mixture. Simmer the picadillo for 45-60 minutes or until the potatoes are softened.

Tips

Try adding jalapeño peppers to the picadillo for added heat and flavor.

90. Classic Tuna Macaroni Salad

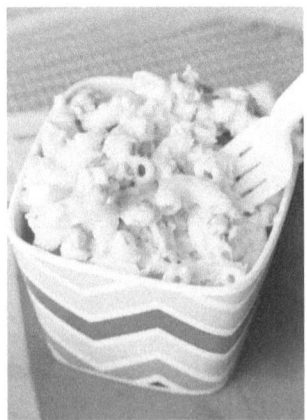

Summary

There is probably nothing better than to be able to treat ourselves with chilled tuna macaroni salad. No fancy ingredients added in the recipe – it's a budget-friendly classic version, which you can alter as per your needs.

Ingredients

- 2 cups elbow macaroni
- 2 cans tuna, drained
- 1 ½ cups mayonnaise
- Salt, to taste
- 4 hardboiled eggs
- 1 can peas, drained
- Black pepper, to taste

Method

1. Cook macaroni according to package instructions. Mix all other ingredients with macaroni. Chill and serve the salad.

Tips

You can turn this regular salad into something fancier by adding vegetables and seasonings of your choice.

91. Shrimp, Avocado and Grapefruit Salad

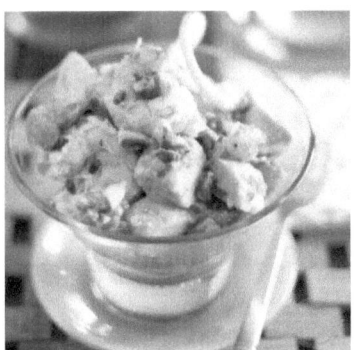

Summary

Simple and extremely easy, this nutritious salad recipe is not only healthy but is also highly comforting. Costing just a little above $1 per serving, you will be able to whip-up this comforting salad any day of the week.

Ingredients

- 12 oz. shrimps, deveined and peeled
- 1 avocado, sliced into 12 wedges

- 2 tablespoons chopped tarragon
- 6 cups romaine lettuce, chopped
- 1 grapefruit, juice extracted while segmenting
- 2 ½ tablespoons olive oil
- 2 teaspoons brown sugar
- ½ teaspoon salt
- 1/4th teaspoon black pepper

Method

1. Season shrimps with 1/4th teaspoon salt and 1/8th teaspoon pepper. Cook shrimps in 1½ tablespoons of oil in a pan for 3-4 minutes. Set aside. Combine grapefruit juice with remaining salt, olive oil, tarragon, remaining pepper, brown sugar and lettuce and toss to combine. Arrange lettuce mixture on plates. Top with shrimps and grapefruit sections. Serve.

Tips

You can also grill the shrimps for adding a punch of intense flavor to the salad.

92. Korean Fish Stir Fry

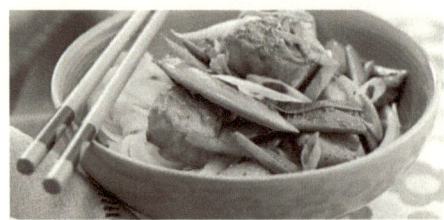

Summary

There is probably no better and easier means of including nutritious fish in your daily diet than to opt for this healthy and easy-to-prepare stir-fry recipe. It also surprisingly fits the budget of $10.

Ingredients

- 12.34 oz. Basa fish fillets, cubed
- 3.5 oz. sugar snap peas, trimmed
- 8.8 oz. cooked rice noodles
- 2 tablespoons soy sauce
- 1 tablespoon rice wine

- 1 red bell pepper, sliced
- 2 garlic cloves, crushed
- 4 green onions, finely chopped
- 1 small red chili, seeded
- 2 tablespoons oil

Method

1. Combine sesame oil, rice wine, soy sauce, chili and garlic in a bowl. Set aside. Stir-fry the fish cubes in 2 tablespoons of oil for 2 minutes. Add snap peas, bell pepper and onion. Stir fry for another 2-3 minutes. Pour rice wine sauce over vegetables. Stir fry for another 1-2 minutes, until sauce thickens. Serve everything over cooked noodles.

Tips

You can also cook the dish with other types of noodles, if you don't get rice noodles.

93. Seafood Skewers

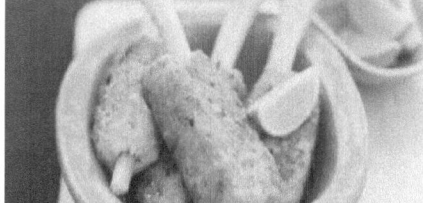

Summary

Great to serve at parties and even at home, you can fit these seafood skewers in your budget pretty easily.

Ingredients

- 16 oz. large shrimps, peeled and deveined
- 4 tablespoons chili sauce
- 8 sea scallops
- 2 garlic cloves
- 4 tablespoons olive oil
- ½ teaspoon red pepper sauce

- Cooked rice
- Black pepper

Method

1. Marinade shrimps and scallops in olive oil, chili sauce, hot pepper sauce, garlic and pepper in fridge for 1 hour. Discard the marinade and thread shrimps and scallops in iron skewers. Grill covered for 5 minutes on each side over medium heat. Serve the skewers over warm rice.

Tips

Substitute chili sauce and hot pepper sauce to barbecue sauce, if you want a milder flavor for these kebobs.

94. Tuna Noodle Casserole

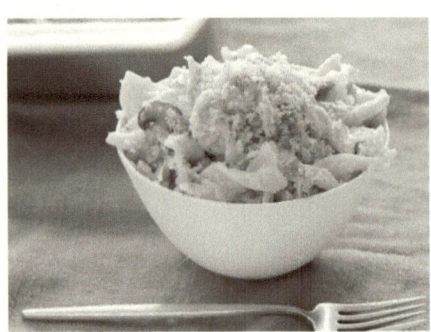

Summary

Popular among both kids and elders, this gorgeous and supremely healthy tuna noodle casserole will consume just about $7-8 of your budget and a few minutes of your time to get prepared.

Ingredients

- 9 oz. tuna
- 8 oz. sea shell pasta, cooked
- ½ cup shredded cheddar cheese
- ½ cup sour cream
- 3/4th cup green peas
- 11 oz. cream of mushroom soup, diluted
- ½ cup milk

Method

1. Mix mushroom soup, milk and sour cream. Toss the pasta in sour cream mixture. Add peas and tuna and toss again. Transfer noodles to a greased casserole dish and bake covered in a 375 degrees Fahrenheit oven for 25 minutes. Spread cheese on top of casserole after 5 minutes and bake uncovered for an extra 5 minutes or until the cheese melts. Serve.

Tips

This recipe can be made more interesting and healthier by adding some vegetables of your choice to it, like broccoli, bell peppers etc.

95. White Fish Baked with Lemon Thyme and Garlic

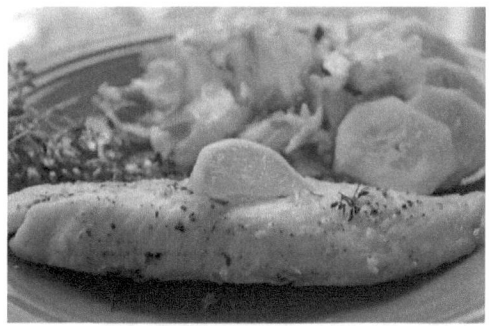

Summary

Want a dose of omega-3 fatty acids and proteins in your diet without indulging in anything too fancy and heavy? Try this easy fish recipe that serves 4-6 people under $10.

Ingredients

- 4 4-oz. Tilapia fish filets
- Juice of ¼th lemon
- 1 ½ tablespoons butter
- 2 tablespoons crushed garlic
- 1 teaspoon lemon rind
- Handful of lemon thyme sprigs
- Salt, to taste
- Pepper, to taste

Method

1. Melt butter with garlic, lemon rind and lemon juice. Pour that into a baking pan. Place half lemon thyme sprigs and seasoned fish filets over melted butter mixture. Place remaining sprigs over filets. Bake fish in a 400 degrees Fahrenheit preheated oven for 20 minutes. Serve over mashed potatoes or rice.

Tips

Drizzle a bit of lemon juice over fish filets after serving for adding a twist to the flavors.

96. Fettuccine Seafood Alfredo

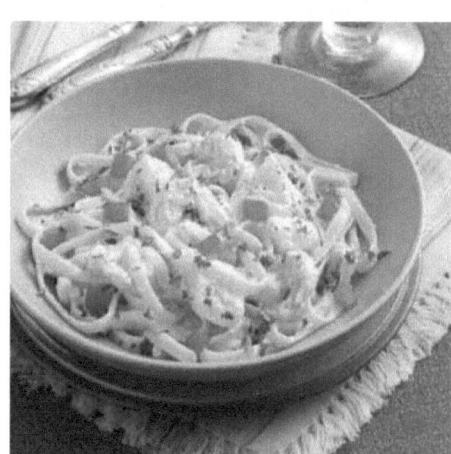

Summary

A classic Italian dish, this elegant seafood recipe can also be fitted into your budget-diet, if you follow this simple recipe.

Ingredients

- ½ lb. lump crabmeat
- 12 oz. evaporated milk
- 12 oz. uncooked fettuccine pasta
- 4 tablespoons sour cream
- 6 garlic cloves, minced
- 1/4th cup grated parmesan cheese
- 1 lb. uncooked shrimps, peeled and deveined

- 4 tablespoons minced fresh basil
- 2 tablespoons olive oil
- ½ teaspoon salt

Method

1. Cook fettuccine according to the cooking instructions provided on its package. Cook the shrimps in 1 tablespoon of olive oil over medium heat for 3-4 minutes. Set aside.

2. Sauté garlic in remaining oil. Add milk and salt. Bring mixture to boil. Whisk-in sour cream and cheese after removing sauce from heat. Add drained pasta, shrimp and crabmeat to sauce. Heat through and serve.

Tips

You can replace garlic with granulated garlic to make the recipe easier and cheaper.

97. Roasted Mushroom and Lentil Soup

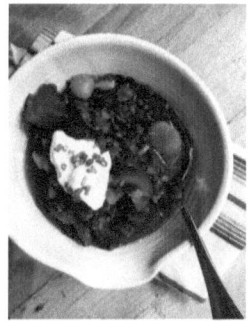

Summary

The rich and spicy flavor of the soup combined with the filling lentils and mushrooms make this soup a heartwarming dinner option, which promises to fit your budget.

Ingredients

- 1 lb. cremini mushrooms, quartered
- 1 shallot, minced
- quart vegetable broth
- 2 celery stalks, minced

- 2 garlic cloves, minced
- ½ cup of uncooked lentils
- 2 tablespoons olive oil

Method

1. Toss mushroom slices with 1 tablespoon of olive oil. Spread in a baking sheet. Roast mushrooms for 15 minutes. Set aside. Cook shallots, celery and garlic in remaining olive oil over medium heat for 5 minutes.

2. Add mushrooms and chicken broth to the vegetables mixture. Stir and let the soup cook for 30 minutes. Add the lentils and cook for another 20 minutes. Serve.

Tips

Serve the soup with a slice of crusty bread to turn it into a hearty and filling meal.

98. Sour Cream and Chives Pasta

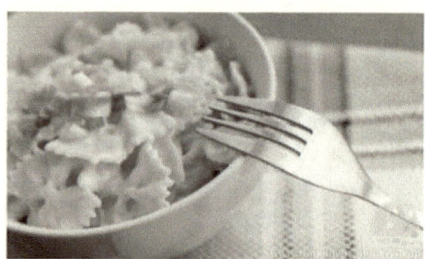

Summary

Perfect for nights when you come back home drained and tired, this delicious sour cream and chives pasta recipe can be whipped-up in just 5-6 minutes and you will be able to nourish yourself with something really tantalizing for just $4-5.

Ingredients

- 1.1 oz. cooked bowtie pasta
- 1 garlic clove, minced
- ½ cup butter
- ½ cup chopped onion
- 3/4th cup sour cream

- 2 tablespoons finely chopped chives
- 4 tablespoons grated cheese
- ½ onion, finely chopped
- 2 tablespoons chopped parsley

Method

1. Combine everything, except pasta in a sauce pan. Cook sauce over low heat for 5 minutes. Toss pasta with sauce, garnish with parsley and serve.

Tips

It is better to freeze the cooked pasta alone without the sauce, as sour cream and fresh herbs may not freeze well. Just thaw frozen cooked pasta and toss with sauce to serve.

99. Black Eyed Peas and Greens

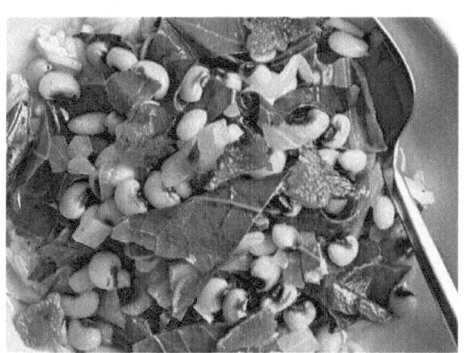

Summary

Loaded with vitamins, calcium, magnesium and other vital nutrients, this kale salad is a fine way of indulging in kale if you refrain yourself from eating raw greens.

Ingredients

- 2 cups cooked black-eyed peas
- 1 ½ lbs. kale, washed and drained
- ½ small sweet onion
- 2 tablespoons apple cider vinegar
- 1 tablespoon chopped garlic

- A pinch of red pepper flakes
- 1 tablespoon olive oil

Method

1. Boil kale in a potful of water until wilted. Drain and set aside. Sauté onions in oil in a skillet. Add garlic and cook for 2 minutes. Add black-eyed peas, salt and pepper flakes. Cook for another 3 minutes. Turn off heat, stir-in kale and vinegar. Serve.

Tips

Blanching the kales will yield crunchier greens.

100. Potato and Broccoli Casserole

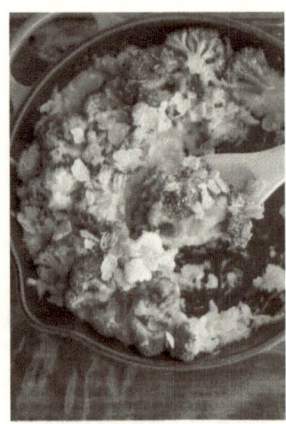

Summary

Made using healthy ingredients and vegetables, this casserole is a fine way of feeding kids some nutritious food. And the great news is you can feed up to 6-8 people under $10 with this dish.

Ingredients

- 10 oz. broccoli florets
- 15 oz. breadcrumbs
- 1 lb. red potato, cubed
- ½ gallon low-fat milk
- 8 oz. shredded low-fat cheddar cheese

Method

1. Boil potatoes in water for 20 minutes or until softened. Reserve 1 cup of cooking liquid, drain the remaining water, reserving a little and set aside the potatoes.

2. Mash potatoes with reserved liquid. Steam broccoli florets according to package instructions. Transfer potato mixture to a greased baking dish and add broccoli and milk. Bake the mixture in a 375 degrees Fahrenheit preheated oven for 35 minutes. Sprinkle breadcrumbs and cheese on top and bake for an additional 5 minutes. Serve once done.

Tips

To retain the crunchiness of the broccoli florets you can blanch those instead of steaming.

101. Vegetarian Tacos

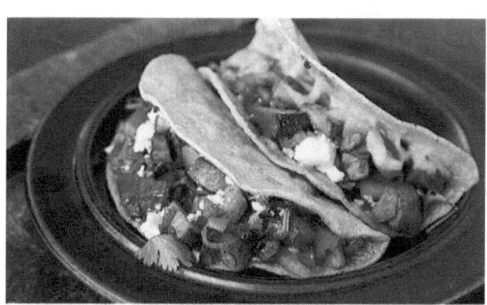

Summary

Spruce up your weekend dinner with these healthy and tasty vegetarian tacos. Filled with good nutrients and loads of proteins, these tacos will fit your budget for serving an entire family.

Ingredients

- 12 oz. chunky salsa
- Shredded Mexican cheese blend
- Taco shells
- 15.5 oz. kidney beans
- 1 head of romaine lettuce, shredded
- A pinch of ground chipotle pepper

Method

1. Rinse and heat-up the kidney beans in a saucepan with chipotle peppers. Heat-up the taco shells. Fill those up with kidney beans, cheese, salsa and lettuce. Serve.

Tips

You can also use dry kidney beans for an organic option. For that, simply soak kidney beans in water for 5-6 hours, drain and heat through for the taco.

102. Parmigiana Allai Melanzane (Eggplant Bake)

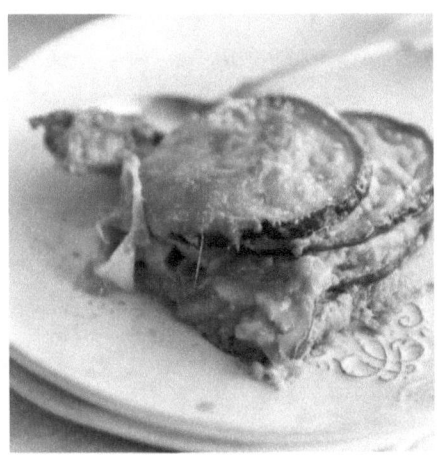

Summary

This eggplant bake recipe makes for a light and healthy dinner dish – one which you will be able to enjoy on a regular basis, without shunning out much of your energy or funds.

Ingredients

- 2 large eggplants, sliced thinly
- 4.4 oz. grated mozzarella cheese
- 2 oz. olive oil
- 2 oz. grated parmesan cheese
- 16.9 oz. pasta sauce
- 1 teaspoon salt
- Black pepper, to taste

Method

1. Sprinkle salt over eggplant slices. Place a bowl over eggplant slices and allow those to stand for 30 minutes, so that eggplant slices weigh down. Rinse under cold water and pat dry. Grill eggplant slices after brushing those with olive oil. Layer half of the eggplant slices in a baking dish and season with pepper.

2. Top with ½ of pasta sauce, ½ of parmesan cheese and ½ of mozzarella cheese. Repeat same process of layering, finishing with cheese. Bake in a 356 degrees Fahrenheit preheated oven for 30 minutes and serve.

Tips

Swipe half of the eggplants with zucchini slices and grill those to add crunch and extra nutrition to the dish.

103. 5-Ingredient Power Casserole

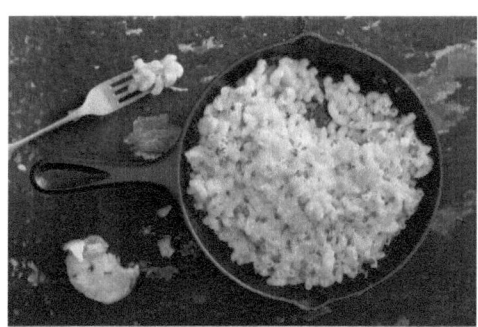

Summary

A simple yet perfect side dish that complements any main dish and yields enough to feed a family for days under just $10, this casserole is really worth-a-try.

Ingredients

- 15 oz. whole corn kernels, drained
- ½ cup melted butter
- 1 cup sour cream
- 8 oz. corn muffin mix
- 15 oz. creamed corn

Method

1. Mix all the ingredients and pour into a greased casserole dish. Bake the casserole uncovered in a 350 degrees Fahrenheit preheated oven for 50-55 minutes.

Tips

You can add hot sauce or a bit of red pepper flakes and salt to add a bit of twist to the flavor of the casserole.

Final Words

I would like to thank you for downloading my book and I hope I have been able to help you and educate you about something new.

If you have enjoyed this book and would like to share your positive thoughts, could you please take 30 seconds of your time to go back and give me a review on my Amazon book page!

I greatly appreciate seeing these reviews because it helps me share my hard work!

Again, thank you and I wish you all the best with your cooking journey!

Last Chance to Get YOUR Bonus!

FOR A LIMITED TIME ONLY – Get Olivia's best-selling book *"The #1 Cookbook: Over 170+ of the Most Popular Recipes Across 7 Different Cuisines!"* absolutely FREE!

Readers have absolutely loved this book because of the wide variety of recipes. It is highly recommended you check these recipes out and see what you can add to your home menu!

Once again, as a big thank-you for downloading this book, I'd like to offer it to you *100% FREE for a LIMITED TIME ONLY!*

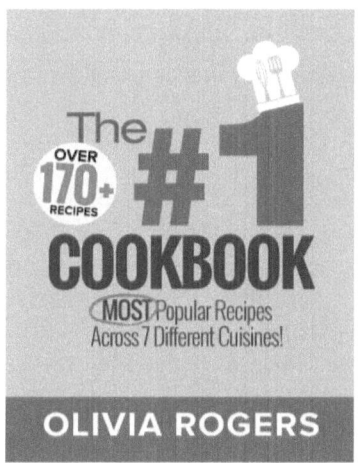

Get your free copy at:

TheMenuAtHome.com/Bonus

Disclaimer

This book and related site provides recipe and food advice in an informative and educational manner only, with information that is general in nature and that is not specific to you, the reader. The contents of this book and related site are intended to assist you and other readers in your personal efforts. Consult your physician or nutritionist regarding the applicability of any information provided in our information to you.

Nothing in this book should be construed as personal advice or diagnosis, and must not be used in this manner. The information provided about conditions is general in nature. This information does not cover all possible uses, actions, precautions, side-effects, or interactions of medicines, or medical procedures. The information in this site should not be considered as complete and does not cover all diseases, ailments, physical conditions, or their treatment.

No Warranties: The authors and publishers don't guarantee or warrant the quality, accuracy, completeness, timeliness, appropriateness or suitability of the information in this book, or of any product or services referenced by this site.

The information in this site is provided on an "as is" basis and the authors and publishers make no representations or warranties of any kind with respect to this information. This site may contain inaccuracies, typographical errors, or other errors.

Liability Disclaimer: The publishers, authors, and other parties involved in the creation, production, provision of information, or delivery of this site specifically disclaim any responsibility, and shall not be held liable for any damages, claims, injuries, losses, liabilities, costs, or obligations including any direct, indirect, special, incidental, or consequences damages (collectively known as "Damages") whatsoever and howsoever caused, arising out of, or in connection with the use or misuse of the site and the information contained within it, whether such Damages arise in contract, tort, negligence, equity, statute law, or by way of other legal theory.

www.ingramcontent.com/pod-product-compliance
Lightning Source LLC
Chambersburg PA
CBHW031127080526
44587CB00011B/1139